DR. SEBI'S ALKALINE HERBS

Discover the Alkaline Herbal Path for Full-Body Detox and Lifelong Health. | Cleansing Teas, Infusions and Decoctions for Natural Healing

ROSALINDA MONTES

DR. SEBI'S ALKALINE HERBS

Discover the Alkaline Herbal Path for Full-Body Detox and Lifelong Health. | Cleansing Teas, Infusions and Decoctions for Natural Healing

CONTENTS

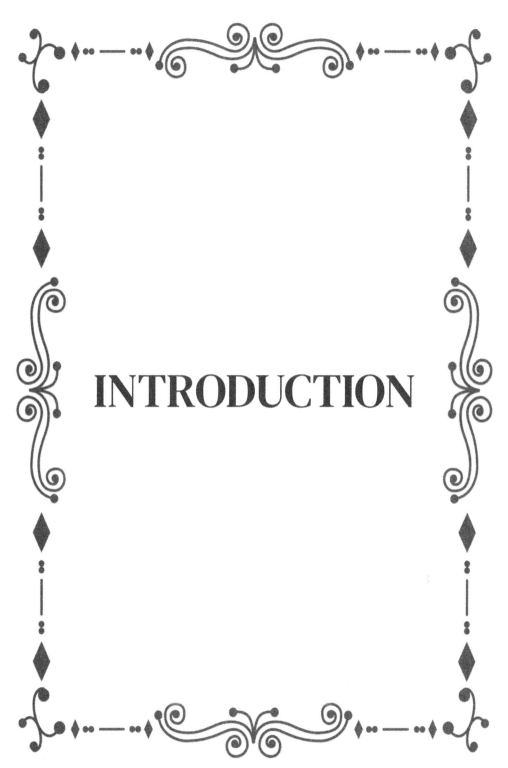

INTRODUCTION

Developing An Understanding of Dr. Sebi's Philosophy

Dr. Sebi, born Alfredo Bowman, was a renowned biochemist, pathologist, herbalist, and naturalist. Hailing from Honduras, he committed his whole life to developing a more in-depth understanding of the thorough potential bond between humans and nature, mainly focusing on the healing powers that some foods and herbs hold towards our bodies and health. Indeed, at the heart of Dr. Sebi's philosophy, there is a firm belief that our body can generate self-healing reactions, which could be triggered through a diet of alkaline, unprocessed, and plant-based foods.

The critical concept lying behind Dr. Sebi's approach is the notion of cellular food. According to his understanding, diseases manifest themselves once our body's cells become toxic due to our consumption of harmful or acidic foods. Therefore, he highlights how we can re-establish our bodies' natural vitality and health by consuming alkaline, natural, and "electric" foods. The healing herbs recommended within Dr. Sebi's alkaline diet own unique medical features, as they were frequently sourced from the genuine landscapes of the Caribbean, Central and South America, and Africa.

To summarize, Dr. Sebi's beliefs and claims pivot on following an alkaline diet, which embodies herbs, seeds, nuts, grains, vegetables and fruits into one's eating habits to arouse an alkaline effect within the body's pH level. This whole concept of food consumption diverges entirely from the Western diet's standards, which revolve around artificial additives, processed foods, and toxins. On the other hand, it is deliberately designed to diminish inflammation, eliminate harmful toxins, and establish a favourable environment for the body's innate healing mechanisms.

Dr. Sebi's wisdom and teachings have been precious, profound, and life-changing. His notions encourage us to avoid contemporary diets that negatively affect our bodies and the environment. Instead, they urge us to embrace the ancient wisdom of the Earth, just as our ancestors did. By doing this, he presents a way that guarantees good health and brings the opportunity for healing, revitalization, and a truly fulfilling life.

As we further delve deeper into this book, we will unfold the details of Dr. Sebi's philosophy, the astonishing benefits of alkaline herbs, and the path toward a vibrant and healthy life.

The Value of An Alkaline Herbal Path

A leading pillar of Dr. Sebi's philosophy revolves around the alkaline herbal approach, which promotes the intake of specific herbs and plant-based foods that help to create an alkaline environment within our bodies. The notion of 'alkalinity' concerns the pH level of our body's fluids and tissues, ranging from 0 (highly acidic) to 14 (highly alkaline), with 7 being the neutral point.

The pH level of our body is essential to preserve our homeostasis process, as well as our overall health. Although the pH levels in different parts of our body may differ, our blood pH is carefully regulated within a range of 7.35 to 7.45, which is slightly alkaline. Hence, if our body's pH deviates much from these values, it can lead to health conditions such as weakened immune function, fatigue, and even more severe ailments like cardiovascular diseases and diabetes.

The conventional Western diet, which incorporates refined sugars, meats, and processed food, often triggers high acidity levels within our bodies, interfering with our pH balance. Contrarily, Dr. Sebi's natural approach to nutrition through an alkaline herbal path focuses on consuming whole plant-based foods that have an alkaline effect on our bodies. By incorporating these foods into our daily intake, we can help our body to enhance our overall well-being, preserving an appropriate pH balance and strengthening our system against diseases.

The herbal remedies and plant-based foods Dr. Sebi supports are rich in minerals, phytochemicals, and antioxidants that provide us with fundamental nourishments to boost our immune system, also optimizing our metabolic functions. Indeed, embracing the alkaline herbal path goes far beyond committing to a diet; instead, it is about adopting a lifestyle that completely aligns with human biology and nature principles. By all means, it is a holistic transformation through how we develop a more in-depth perception of our body's well-being and connection with the environment.

Advantages Of Undergoing a Full-Body Detox

D r. Sebi emphasizes the concept of full-body detoxification, as he firmly believes it is essential to support our health and well-being. This method involves removing substances or toxins that gradually build up in our bodies due to lifestyle decisions, eating habits, and exposure to pollutants. By undergoing the process of detoxification, we can restore our body functions, regain energy, and establish an adequate foundation for overall long-term well-being.

Dr. Sebi firmly suggests a regular detoxification process, considering it a natural mechanism for the body to reset itself. Let's explore some of the advantages linked to body detoxification:

1. Enhanced organs' functionality: Supporting the body's cleansing system, detoxification aids the main organs responsible for this process, such as the lungs, the kidneys, the liver, and the skin. By getting rid of toxins, these organs can perform thoroughly, enhancing the body's well-being and health.

2. Boosted energy levels: When harmful substances accumulate in our bodies, it can result in chronic tiredness and lack of energy. A detoxification process can assist you in revitalizing your body, enhancing energy levels and promoting mental and physical capabilities.

3. Improvement of the immune system's strength: There are several benefits in detoxifying your body, including boosting your immune system's resistance. Indeed, when the toxin load within the body is reduced, the immune system works effectively, protecting our body from infections and diseases. Moreover, plenty of alkaline herbs employed in detoxification contain nutrients that can further bolster our bodily functions.

4. Enhanced digestion: A thorough detoxification of the body can aid in purifying the digestive tract, alleviating symptoms like constipation, excessive gas, bloating, and other common digestive problems. This, in turn, promotes the enhanced absorption of nutrients and fosters a healthier and more balanced gut flora.

5. Weight control: Detoxification can significantly help you to manage and shed weight by enhancing the body's metabolism and curbing cravings for unhealthy aliments.

6. Mental clarity: Toxins can negatively impact brain functions. A considerable amount of people mentioned they experienced an improvement in their concentration and mental clarity after undergoing a detoxification process.

7. Improved Skin Health: By eliminating substances that contribute to skin problems, like eczema, acne, and premature aging, a detoxification process can result in more healthful and vibrant skin.

According to this, full-body detoxification represents a crucial step to rejuvenate your body and set the path towards healthier living. By using the alkaline herbs recommended by Dr. Sebi during this process, you will either help your body to eliminate toxins or provide yourself with essential nutrients able to support your body's natural healing capabilities. In the following sections, we will explore the concept of detoxification and how you can seamlessly integrate it into your wellness routine.

Lifelong Health: A Consistent Journey

According to Dr. Sebi, health goes far beyond the mere concept of being free from illness. On the other hand, it embodies our whole mental, physical, and social well-being. It is about attaining a state of vitality, a life filled with energy, vibrancy and strength. Dr. Sebi believes that the journey towards lasting health and vitality starts by acknowledging nature's potential healing and rejuvenating powers on our bodies.

Incorporating alkaline foods and herbs represents, indeed, a benchmark in achieving long-term health advantages, such as increased energy levels, improved mood and digestion, and a reduced likelihood of developing chronic illnesses like diabetes, heart disease, and cancer.

By ensuring the body's pH remains balanced, these herbs and foods support our body in creating an environment that promotes the optimal functioning of our organs and cells.

Moreover, the alkaline herbal approach contributes to our holistic well-being, a key aspect of our overall health, as maintaining vitality throughout our life goes above and beyond our physical state. Indeed, it also entails nurturing a balanced mental and emotional state. Numerous herbs and plant-based foods have been discovered to promote acuity while alleviating anxiety, stress, and depression.

Embracing the alkaline herbal approach represents a transition towards mindful eating, which entails being engaged in the present while enjoying our meals and valuing the nourishment they provide us. This awareness practice can improve our connection with the aliments we eat daily, minimizing the likelihood of overeating and fostering healthier ideas of our bodies.

Finally, following the alkaline path also strengthens our bond with nature. Cultivating your herbs, for instance, grants you access to chemical-free ingredients to integrate into your meals and allows you to engage with the environment. This process has been associated with boosting individuals' mental health in several studies.

In our discovery of alkaline herbs and the teachings of Dr. Sebi, this book will act as a companion on your path to a vibrant and healthy life. It is about embracing a way of living that nourishes your spirit and brings peace to your mind and body.

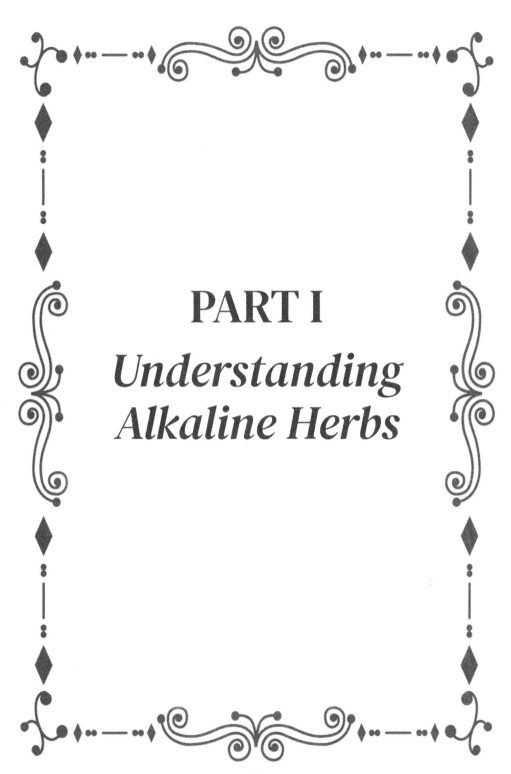

PART I

Understanding Alkaline Herbs

Mastering The Concept of Alkaline Herbs

To truly grasp the realm of alkaline herbs, it is fundamental to comprehend the defining peculiarities of what makes an herb "alkaline." The concept itself is based on the pH scale, which gauges a substance's alkalinity levels or acidity. This scale spans from 0 to 14, with 0 representing the highest level of acidity, 14 the highest level of alkalinity, and 7 being a state of neutrality.

The idea of alkaline herbs is closely related to the concept of the alkaline diet. This particular eating plan encourages the intake of foods that are thought to have an alkalizing effect on the body's pH balance. The underlying belief is that our dietary choices can significantly influence our body's pH level and consequently impact our overall well-being.

Therefore, alkaline herbs are a type of herbs that, once ingested, promote an alkaline state within the body. These herbs are rich in minerals such as magnesium, potassium, iron, zinc, and calcium. On the other hand, they are relatively low in phosphorus, chloride, and sulfur, which can leave behind a residue within our bodies.

Considering this concept from a biochemical perspective, the nourishing properties found in alkaline herbs support the balance of the acidity levels within our bloodstream. This, in turn, promote an alkaline state, which is widely recognized as beneficial for the optimal functioning of our body's cells.

However, it is worth mentioning that not every herb owns alkaline properties. Interestingly enough, the pH level of a plant does not necessarily indicate whether it will have an alkaline impact on our body. Otherwise, what truly matters is the mineral composition of the herb, as well as how our bodies metabolize it. Dr. Sebi focused extensively on incorporating alkaline herbs into his healing approach as he believed they could eliminate toxins, restore the body, and promote an elevated state of health.

Throughout this book, we will further explore the alkaline herbs Dr. Sebi endorsed, their various health advantages, and ways you can seamlessly include them in your meals. However, before we delve into those specifics, let's closely examine alkaline herbs' benefits and why they play such a crucial role in achieving holistic well-being and vitality.

The Health Benefits Brought by Alkaline Herbs

As previously mentioned, herbs with alkaline properties provide several advantages that boost our overall well-being. Their effects extend further to adjusting our body's pH levels and substantially contribute to preventing diseases. Some of the health advantages alkaline herbs provide are the following:

1. Reduced inflammation and weight management

Excessive and chronic inflammation can trigger various health issues, such as cancer, heart disease, and arthritis. Several alkaline herbs, such as cuachalalate, burdock root, and blue vervain, own anti-inflammatory properties. Incorporating these herbs into your routine can assist you in managing your body's inflammation. Certain herbs with alkaline properties can also aid in managing weight. They can enhance our metabolism, generating a feeling of fullness and, therefore, curb cravings for unhealthy aliments. These herbs are commonly used to assist individuals with their weight-loss goals.

2. Improved immune functions and digestive health:

Alkaline herbs are known for their antioxidants and essential nutrients, which fortifies our immune system. Having an efficient immune system is vital to generate protection against illnesses. Herbs like elderberry and echinacea are widely known for their immune-boosting properties. Moreover, herbs with alkaline properties are also known for containing rich amounts of dietary fibres, which are essential for our body's digestive well-being. These herbs can aid in maintaining regular bowel movements, as well as the equilibrium of gut flora, preventing constipation and other digestive problems.

3. Enhanced mental well-being, body detoxification, and energy levels

There are a variety of herbs that have been discovered to support mental wellness. They can help you alleviate anxiety and stress and facilitate sleep. Furthermore, these herbs can also enhance the body's natural detoxification processes, as they purify the blood, facilitating optimal liver performance and aiding the kidneys in filtering toxins. Indeed, renowned alkaline herbs, like muicle, dandelion, and burdock, have great detoxifying qualities. Lastly, the regular incorporation of alkaline herbs within your daily food intake can boost your energy levels, as these herbs can potentially improve the absorption of nutrients and enhance our cellular function, increasing vitality.

The abovementioned advantages illustrate how alkaline herbs can contribute to our well-being.

In the next chapter, you will find information about Dr. Sebi's authorized alkaline herbs, including their specific benefits and recommended uses.

Dr. Sebi's Approved Alkaline Herbs

This guide provides an overview of all alkaline herbs approved by Dr. Sebi, highlighting their benefits, cultivation, sourcing, preparation, usage, storing and preservation.

Bladderwrack: The Seaside Marvel

Bladderwrack, scientifically named Fucus vesiculosus, is a type of seaweed found on the coasts of the North Sea, the Atlantic, and the Pacific Oceans. Endorsed by Dr. Sebi, this sea vegetable has a wealth of health benefits and applications, making it a fantastic addition to an alkaline lifestyle.

Health Benefits:

A rich source of iodine, Bladderwrack is often utilized for thyroid health. The iodine present in this seaweed stimulates thyroid activity, ensuring the healthy production of hormones that regulate various essential body functions.

It is also known for its anti-inflammatory properties, making it a go-to herb for conditions like arthritis and gout. The rich mineral content, including calcium, magnesium, and potassium, can contribute to bone health, reducing the risk of osteoporosis.

Another noteworthy property of Bladderwrack is its potential in aiding weight loss. This herb is high in fiber, which aids digestion and promotes feelings of fullness, helping to manage overeating.

Cultivation and Sourcing:

As a sea vegetable, Bladderwrack is harvested from the ocean rather than cultivated in a traditional sense. It's crucial to source Bladderwrack from clean and unpolluted waters to avoid harmful substances like heavy metals.

Preparation and Usage:

Bladderwrack is often consumed in a powdered or encapsulated form, but it can also be steeped to make a beneficial tea. Start with small amounts and monitor your body's reaction to adjust the dosage as needed.

Storage and Preservation:

Bladderwrack, like most herbs, should be stored in a cool, dark place, away from direct sunlight. If you have Bladderwrack in its raw form, it can be dried and stored for long-term use. Powdered or encapsulated Bladderwrack should be kept in an airtight container to preserve its potency.

A marine gift of nature, Bladderwrack offers a unique and potent blend of health benefits. Its nutritional profile and broad spectrum of applications make it a standout in Dr. Sebi's collection of approved herbs. The inclusion of this herb in your journey towards optimal health signifies your commitment to embracing the richness and variety that nature has to offer.

Blue Vervain: The Nervine Powerhouse

Blue Vervain, scientifically known as Verbena hastata, is a potent herb recognized for its diverse healing properties. It's one of the prized constituents of Dr. Sebi's herbal arsenal due to its alkaline nature and its ability to support various aspects of health. This chapter aims to delve into the intricacies of this versatile herb, exploring its benefits, cultivation and sourcing, preparation, and usage guidelines.

Native to North America, Blue Vervain is a perennial plant that thrives in sunny locales with abundant moisture. Its thin, elegant stalks topped with small lavender-blue flowers make it a captivating sight in wild meadows and grasslands. But, the charm of Blue Vervain is not only in its beauty; it's within the potent phytochemicals found in its stems, leaves, and flowers.

Health Benefits:

Blue Vervain is categorized as a nervine herb, meaning it possesses properties that significantly benefit the nervous system. It's known for its calming effects, and has been traditionally used to alleviate stress, anxiety, and insomnia. This herb also works as a potent analgesic and anti-inflammatory agent, often used to soothe headaches, muscle pain, and arthritis symptoms.

Additionally, Blue Vervain supports digestion, easing indigestion, bloating, and constipation. Its expectorant properties help clear mucus from the lungs, making it a useful herb for respiratory issues such as bronchitis and asthma.

Cultivation and Sourcing:

As Blue Vervain prefers a sunny habitat with moist, well-drained soil, sourcing from areas mimicking these conditions ensures the best quality. It's crucial to remember that the growing environment significantly impacts the quality and potency of herbs.

When sourcing Blue Vervain, look for organically grown or wildcrafted plants. Suppliers should be transparent about their cultivation practices, ensuring no chemical pesticides or fertilizers have been used. High-quality Blue Vervain should have a vibrant color, a distinct aroma, and should be free from mold or any signs of decay.

Preparation and Usage:

To tap into the benefits of Blue Vervain, it's commonly used in the form of tea or tincture. For tea, simply steep one to two teaspoons of the dried herb in hot water for about 10-15 minutes, then strain and enjoy. As a tincture, the dosage generally lies between 2-4 ml, taken three times a day. However, it's important to remember that dosage might vary based on individual needs and it's always advisable to consult a professional before starting a new regimen.

Preserving and Storing:

To maintain its potency, Blue Vervain should be stored correctly. Keep it in an airtight container, in a cool, dark place. Properly stored, the dried herb can last for about a year.

Burdock Root: The Blood Purifier

Burdock Root, recognized scientifically as Arctium lappa, is a staple in Dr. Sebi's approved herbs. Known for its blood purifying and skin healing properties, burdock root is a powerful herb that supports holistic health and well-being.

Health Benefits:

The health benefits of burdock root are extensive. It is a potent antioxidant, helping to neutralize harmful free radicals in the body. This, in turn, reduces inflammation and may slow the aging process.

One of burdock root's most renowned benefits is its blood purifying property. It's believed to cleanse the bloodstream of toxins, thus promoting overall health. This cleansing action also has a profound effect on skin health, and it's often used to help alleviate skin conditions such as acne, eczema, and psoriasis.

Moreover, burdock root supports healthy digestion due to its high dietary fiber content. It aids in maintaining a healthy gut and may alleviate common digestive ailments. Furthermore, it is known to maintain healthy kidney and liver function, ensuring these organs' optimal operation.

Cultivation and Sourcing:

Burdock is a hardy biennial plant that is grown worldwide but is native to Northern Europe and Asia. It thrives in well-drained, fertile soil, and under full to partial sunlight.

For therapeutic use, ensure that you source your burdock root from a reliable supplier, guaranteeing that it's grown organically and harvested sustainably. Wild harvested burdock can be found, but care should be taken to ensure it's collected responsibly and from a clean, unpolluted area.

Preparation and Usage:

Burdock root can be consumed in several ways. It can be steeped into a tea, made into a tincture, or used in cooking. Its earthy and sweet flavor makes it a pleasant addition to many dishes. It's important to follow Dr. Sebi's recommended dosage for therapeutic use and to monitor individual responses to adjust dosage accordingly.

Storage and Preservation:

Fresh burdock root should be stored in the refrigerator where it can last for several weeks. Dried burdock root should be kept in an airtight container in a cool, dark, and dry place where it can stay potent for up to a year.

Incorporating burdock root into your herbal regimen can have a profound impact on your health and well-being. Its potent purifying and healing properties make it a powerful ally in pursuing holistic health, in line with Dr. Sebi's vision.

Cascara Sagrada: The Gentle Digestive Tonic

Cascara Sagrada, scientifically known as Rhamnus purshiana, is a well-regarded herb in Dr. Sebi's list of approved herbs. Known for its beneficial effects on the digestive system, this herb has been used for centuries in traditional medicine and continues to be valued in modern herbalism.

Health Benefits:

The most prominent benefit of Cascara Sagrada is its role as a natural laxative. It contains compounds called anthraquinones that stimulate the intestines, helping to ease constipation. As such, it can be a gentle solution for those struggling with irregular bowel movements.

Furthermore, Cascara Sagrada is believed to improve the function of the gallbladder and liver, organs pivotal to the digestive process. This dual action makes the herb a valuable aid in the maintenance of a healthy digestive system.

Cultivation and Sourcing:

Cascara Sagrada is a species of buckthorn native to western North America. It flourishes in moist, well-drained soils and requires a cool, shady environment for optimal growth. When sourcing Cascara Sagrada, it is important to ensure that it is organically grown, free from harmful chemicals or additives that could compromise its health benefits.

Preparation and Usage:

Typically, Cascara Sagrada is used in its dried, aged form. The bark is harvested, dried for at least one year, and then used to prepare herbal remedies. The aging process is critical as fresh Cascara Sagrada can cause severe abdominal cramping.

To consume, Cascara Sagrada is commonly taken as a capsule or used to prepare a tea. The dose should be carefully managed, starting with a low dose and increasing as necessary to avoid potential side effects such as abdominal cramping or diarrhea.

Storage and Preservation:

Proper storage is key to maintaining the effectiveness of Cascara Sagrada. Keep it in a cool, dark, and dry place, preferably in an airtight container. This will help protect the herb from moisture and light, which can deteriorate its quality over time.

Cascara Sagrada is a powerful herb that, when used correctly, can provide relief from digestive discomfort and promote regularity. As a gentle and natural solution to common digestive issues, it embodies Dr. Sebi's philosophy of achieving health and well-being through natural, alkaline herbs. As you integrate this herb into your wellness routine, you are truly embracing a path towards holistic health and vitality.

Chamomile: A Soothing Herb for Health and Serenity

Chamomile, also known as Matricaria chamomilla or Chamaemelum nobile, is a precious member of Dr. Sebi's approved herb list. Renowned for its soothing and calming properties, this dainty flower is not only beautiful but also a powerful ally for your health.

Health Benefits:

Known for its calming properties, chamomile is often used to alleviate stress and promote sleep. It contains apigenin, an antioxidant that binds to certain receptors in your brain that may promote sleepiness and reduce insomnia.

Besides, chamomile is also reputed for its digestive benefits. It may relieve dyspepsia, nausea, and gas, thus making it a good post-meal beverage. Its antispasmodic properties may ease menstrual cramps, and its anti-inflammatory qualities can aid in managing symptoms of osteoarthritis.

Cultivation and Sourcing:

Chamomile is native to Western Europe, India, and western Asia but has been successfully cultivated in various parts of the world. This herb flourishes best in cool conditions and should be planted under full sunlight in well-draining soil. If you're sourcing chamomile, ensure it's from organic, non-GMO sources to guarantee the best quality and efficacy.

Preparation and Usage:

Chamomile tea is the most common way to consume this herb, and it's a delightful experience. The tea has a mild sweetness with hints of apple and earthiness, making it a relaxing and comforting drink.

While it's generally safe to consume, some people may have allergic reactions to chamomile, especially those who are allergic to daisy or ragweed. It's always prudent to test a small amount first or consult a healthcare provider if you're unsure.

Storage and Preservation:

If you've decided to grow your own chamomile, you'll want to know how to store it properly. Fresh chamomile should be used immediately, but it can be dried for long-term storage. To dry chamomile, hang the flowers upside down in a cool, dry, and dark place. Once completely dry, store it in airtight containers and keep them away from direct sunlight and heat to maintain their quality.

Cuachalalate: The Forgotten Wonder of Nature

Cuachalalate, scientifically named Amphipterygium adstringens, is a lesser known but exceptionally potent herb approved by Dr. Sebi.

Cuachalalate is a tree native to Mexico and parts of Central America. Its bark is the most valued part, rich with various medicinal properties. For centuries, this herb has been utilized by indigenous cultures for treating a range of ailments.

Health Benefits:

Known for its potent anti-inflammatory and antimicrobial properties, Cuachalalate is primarily used in managing conditions like gastritis and ulcers. Its astringent qualities make it beneficial in wound healing and reducing bleeding. Moreover, it has been used in traditional medicine to address issues related to the liver and kidneys.

Interestingly, recent scientific investigations have been exploring Cuachalalate's potential in cancer treatments, specifically its effects on reducing tumor growth. While these studies are still in the early stages, they offer exciting possibilities for the medicinal applications of this herb.

Cultivation and Sourcing:

Cuachalalate trees grow well in tropical and subtropical climates, preferring areas with well-draining soils. If you're sourcing Cuachalalate, look for suppliers who ensure sustainable harvesting practices, respecting the life cycle of the tree and promoting the health of the ecosystem.

Preparation and Usage:

The bark of the Cuachalalate tree can be used to prepare teas, infusions, and tinctures. Due to its potent nature, it is advised to begin with small doses, gradually increasing as your body acclimates. Always listen to your body's signals and consult a health professional if in doubt.

Storage and Preservation:

The bark should be stored in a cool, dry place, away from direct sunlight. It's best to keep it in an airtight container to maintain its potency and freshness. If you choose to powder the bark, ensure it's stored in a dark container to protect it from light, which can degrade its therapeutic properties over time.

Cuachalalate, with its significant health-boosting properties, stands as a testament to Dr. Sebi's wisdom in promoting nature's bounty for healing and wellbeing. While relatively lesser-known, this herb holds untapped potential for those on their journey towards an alkaline lifestyle. Embracing the benefits of Cuachalalate, we continue to honor Dr. Sebi's legacy and further our commitment to natural health.

Chaparral: The Resilient Healer of the Desert

Chaparral, scientifically known as Larrea tridentata, is one of Dr. Sebi's cherished alkaline herbs, celebrated for its extraordinary health benefits and healing properties. This chapter ventures into the realm of Chaparral, exploring its health advantages, cultivation and sourcing recommendations, and usage guidelines.

Hailing from the arid regions of the Southwestern United States and Mexico, Chaparral thrives under the burning sun, withstanding harsh climatic conditions that few plants can endure. Its resilience translates into a powerful, natural remedy that can fortify our own bodies in numerous ways.

Health Benefits:

Chaparral is a powerhouse of antioxidants, particularly nordihydroguaiaretic acid (NDGA), known for its potent anti-inflammatory, antiviral, and antibacterial properties. It has been traditionally used by Native American tribes for a variety of ailments, including respiratory conditions, skin disorders, and digestive issues.

Recent studies suggest that Chaparral may inhibit the growth of cancer cells, a promising finding that warrants further investigation. Moreover, it's been used to alleviate symptoms of arthritis and other inflammatory conditions due to its potent anti-inflammatory properties.

Cultivation and Sourcing:

Sourcing Chaparral requires a focus on its natural habitat, as it thrives in desert environments with well-drained soil. If purchasing, ensure that suppliers adhere to sustainable wildcrafting methods. This not only supports the plant's health and potency but also the overall balance and sustainability of the desert ecosystems where Chaparral grows.

Preparation and Usage:

The leaves of the Chaparral plant are the primary part used for medicinal purposes. These can be dried and used to make a strong tea or decoction. When using Chaparral, start with small dosages, monitoring for any possible reactions. While generally safe for most individuals, its potent properties could potentially cause skin reactions or upset stomach in some sensitive individuals.

Storage and Preservation:

Like most herbs, Chaparral should be stored in a cool, dark, and dry place. This can help retain its potent properties for a longer time. You can keep it in an airtight container to prevent contamination and preserve its freshness.

Chaparral stands as a powerful testament to the enduring vitality of nature, even in the most challenging conditions. Its rich history of use in traditional healing practices, coupled with modern scientific insights, make it an important part of the Dr. Sebi's herbal roster. As we incorporate it into our regimen, we're not only tapping into the plant's inherent strength but also connecting with an ancient lineage of herbal wisdom.

Contribo: The Mighty Vine of Wellness

Contribo, or Birthwort, scientifically known as Aristolochia trilobata, is a member of Dr. Sebi's approved herbal list. Originating from Central and South America, it's a vigorous vine, widely utilized in traditional medicine for its potent health benefits.

Health Benefits:

Contribo is often recommended as a general tonic and stimulant, providing a boost to the body's overall well-being. It's reputed to have a positive effect on the digestive system, often used to address issues like indigestion and constipation. Also, Contribo has been applied to manage pain, and it's lauded for its potential anti-inflammatory properties.

Moreover, the plant is thought to be useful in managing conditions such as diabetes, malaria, and snake bites. However, it's crucial to note that these uses are primarily based on traditional practices, and more scientific research is necessary to fully validate these claims.

Cultivation and Sourcing:

Contribo is a tropical plant, flourishing in warm, humid climates. When sourcing, it's vital to ensure the herb's quality. Seek out organic, wild-crafted Contribo, untouched by synthetic chemicals. Traceability is another key factor: suppliers should be able to provide clear information about the plant's origin and the cultivation practices followed.

Preparation and Usage:

Traditionally, Contribo is prepared as a tea or tincture. The herb's potency calls for careful dosage, making it essential to follow guidance from an experienced herbalist. While this mighty vine has shown many beneficial effects, misuse could lead to adverse reactions. Therefore, understanding the proper usage is fundamental.

Storage and Preservation:

Dried Contribo should be stored in a cool, dark place, away from moisture and heat. Keeping the herb in an airtight container will help retain its freshness and potency. As with all herbs, it's best to use it within a specified timeframe for maximum effectiveness.

Dandelion: The Underappreciated Elixir

Dandelion, scientifically known as Taraxacum officinale, is perhaps one of the most underappreciated plants in the botanical world. Often dismissed as a pesky weed, it's a treasure trove of healing properties and is one of the integral elements of Dr. Sebi's approved list of herbs.

Health Benefits:

Dandelion is renowned for its extensive health benefits. Its roots and leaves have been used in traditional medicine for centuries. Rich in antioxidants, it's known to combat inflammation and promote a healthy immune system.

One of the most prominent health benefits of dandelion is its role in promoting liver health. It's often used as a natural detoxifier, assisting the liver in eliminating toxins from the body. Moreover, it supports healthy digestion and can help alleviate minor digestive discomfort.

Additionally, the plant has diuretic properties, which can help increase urine production and reduce water retention. Some preliminary research even suggests that dandelion might help regulate blood sugar and cholesterol levels, although more studies are needed to fully establish these benefits.

Cultivation and Sourcing:

Dandelions are resilient and can grow in a variety of conditions, although they prefer full sunlight and rich, fertile soil. They are commonly found in meadows, lawns, and even cracks in the pavement. However, not all dandelions should be used for consumption, especially those from urban areas or lawns treated with pesticides.

For medicinal use, it's recommended to source dandelions from a reputable supplier who ensures that the plants are grown organically and harvested responsibly.

Preparation and Usage:

Every part of the dandelion – roots, leaves, and flowers – is edible and can be used in different ways. The leaves can be added to salads or steeped into tea, while the roots are often used in herbal infusions or dried and ground as a coffee substitute. The flowers can be used to make wine.

Dr. Sebi's recommended dosage should be adhered to for therapeutic use, and as always, individual responses should be monitored to adjust dosage as needed.

Storage and Preservation:

Fresh dandelion leaves can be stored in the refrigerator, while the roots can be dried and stored in a cool, dark place. Dried dandelion root and leaf, when stored properly, can last for up to a year.

In embracing the dandelion's medicinal qualities, we acknowledge its status as a powerful healing herb rather than a mere weed. Incorporating dandelion into your wellness regimen is a step toward realizing Dr. Sebi's vision of holistic health achieved through nature's bounty.

Elderberry: The Immunity Booster

Elderberry, known scientifically as Sambucus Adoxaceae, is an incredibly beneficial herb treasured by many cultures around the world for its health-promoting qualities. Its popularity soared under Dr. Sebi's recommendations due to its alkaline properties and profound effects on the immune system. This chapter will explore Elderberry in all its aspects, covering its health benefits, cultivation and sourcing details, methods of preparation, and usage guidelines.

Hailing from Europe, Elderberry is a perennial shrub, typically found in sunny, well-drained locations. The plant boasts clusters of tiny white flowers, which ripen into dark, glossy berries during late summer. Its flowers, leaves, bark, and especially berries, are replete with potent compounds that account for its impressive medicinal profile.

Health Benefits:

Elderberry has long been lauded for its immune-boosting qualities. It's rich in antioxidants and vitamins that can help combat inflammation, lower stress, and protect the heart. Most notably, Elderberries are renowned for their antiviral properties. Studies have suggested that Elderberry extract can inhibit the propagation of the influenza virus, shortening flu duration and lessening symptom severity.

Moreover, Elderberries have diuretic, laxative, and detoxifying properties, aiding digestive health and supporting kidney function. They're also traditionally used for alleviating respiratory issues, such as asthma, bronchitis, and sinusitis.

Cultivation and Sourcing:

Elderberries flourish in well-drained, loamy soil under full to partial sun. Sourcing them from regions that replicate these natural conditions will ensure optimal quality. When selecting Elderberries, it's crucial to opt for organically grown or wildcrafted sources. Reputable suppliers should provide clear information about their cultivation practices, confirming the absence of harmful chemical fertilizers or pesticides. High-grade Elderberries should bear a rich color, have a pleasant aroma, and be free from mold or other signs of decay.

Preparation and Usage:

Elderberries can be used in various forms - tea, syrup, or tincture being the most common. To prepare Elderberry tea, steep one tablespoon of dried berries in hot water for 15-20 minutes before straining. For syrup, simmer the berries in water, add a sweetener like agave or date sugar, and let it reduce. The typical tincture dosage ranges from 1-2 ml, taken up to three times a day. As always, it's important to consider individual health circumstances when determining dosage and consult a professional if needed.

Preserving and Storing:

To retain the potency of Elderberries, proper storage is essential. They should be kept in a cool, dark place, inside an airtight container. If preserved correctly, dried Elderberries can last up to a year, maintaining their potency and effectiveness.

Flor de Manita: A Powerful Heart Ally

Flor de Manita, also scientifically known as Chiranthodendron pentadactylon, is one of the lesser-known gems from Dr. Sebi's approved herb list. Hailing from Mexico and Guatemala's high-altitude regions, this distinctive plant, recognized by its hand-shaped flowers, is primarily known for its heart-supporting properties.

Health Benefits:

The most notable attribute of Flor de Manita is its potent cardiovascular benefits. It has been traditionally used in Mexico to manage heart conditions, including arrhythmias, heart failure, and hypertension. It's believed that the plant's bioactive compounds, like flavonoids and tannins, contribute to its heart-protective qualities.

Moreover, Flor de Manita is believed to possess sedative properties, assisting in stress relief and promoting mental tranquility. It is also said to have antispasmodic and analgesic properties, offering relief from muscle spasms and mild discomfort.

Cultivation and Sourcing:

Flor de Manita is a tree that grows in the tropical highlands of Mexico and Guatemala. It thrives best in well-drained, fertile soil, and moderate sunlight. When sourcing Flor de Manita, it's essential to look for suppliers that prioritize sustainable, ethical harvesting practices and ensure the plant's quality and potency are preserved.

Preparation and Usage:

Traditionally, Flor de Manita is prepared as a tea. Its leaves are dried and then steeped in hot water to extract the beneficial compounds. It's crucial to note that the plant is powerful, and usage should be initiated under the guidance of a knowledgeable herbalist or a healthcare provider to ensure appropriate dosing and safety.

Storage and Preservation:

Proper storage is key to maintaining Flor de Manita's potency. The dried leaves should be kept in an airtight container, stored in a cool, dry, and dark place. This will prevent any degradation caused by exposure to light, air, and humidity, thus extending the herb's shelf life.

Gordolobo: The Herbal Champion of Respiratory Health

Gordolobo, otherwise known as Verbascum thapsus or mullein, is an herb that grows abundantly in Europe, North Africa, Asia, and the Americas. Promoted by Dr. Sebi, this herb is celebrated for its rich medicinal properties, particularly in relation to respiratory health.

Health Benefits:

Gordolobo is hailed as an effective herbal remedy for various respiratory ailments, from minor issues such as coughs and sore throats to more severe conditions like bronchitis and asthma. The saponins found in Gordolobo can help loosen mucus, thereby relieving congestion and promoting better respiratory function.

This versatile herb also has potent anti-inflammatory and antiviral properties, which can be beneficial for overall immune health. Additionally, its mucilaginous nature soothes irritated tissues, bringing relief to conditions like gastritis and ulcerative colitis.

Cultivation and Sourcing:

Gordolobo is a hardy plant that thrives in a variety of climates, growing well in both sunny and partially shaded environments. As with other herbs approved by Dr. Sebi, it's essential to source Gordolobo from organic growers who prioritize quality and sustainability in their cultivation practices.

Preparation and Usage:

Gordolobo is often consumed as a tea to alleviate respiratory symptoms. To prepare this, steep the dried leaves and flowers in hot water for about 15 minutes before drinking. Gordolobo can also be found in capsule form, offering a convenient option for daily intake.

Storage and Preservation:

Dried Gordolobo should be stored in a cool, dry place away from direct sunlight to maintain its potency. It can be kept in a sealed glass container to extend its shelf life. As for encapsulated Gordolobo, a closed container is ideal to ensure the capsules remain dry and effective.

With its soothing properties and effectiveness in alleviating respiratory discomfort, Gordolobo is a valuable asset in the collection of Dr. Sebi's recommended herbs. Its gentle action, combined with its potent medicinal properties, serve as a reminder of the incredible healing power of nature. As you incorporate Gordolobo into your lifestyle, you embrace the wisdom of traditional herbal practices, nurturing your body towards optimal health.

Irish Sea Moss: The Superfood from the Sea

Among the most potent and valued plants in Dr. Sebi's arsenal of alkaline foods, Irish Sea Moss, also known as Chondrus crispus, holds a place of distinction. Belonging to the red algae family, it's praised for its rich mineral content and health benefits. This chapter delves deep into the details of Irish Sea Moss, shedding light on its health advantages, sourcing and preparation guidelines, and appropriate usage.

A native to the Atlantic coastlines of North America and Europe, Irish Sea Moss thrives in the rocky regions of the ocean shore. The sea vegetable is marked by its vibrant color, ranging from a yellowish, greenish to purplish, dark red hue, and its unique, leaf-like structure.

Health Benefits:

What truly sets Irish Sea Moss apart is its extraordinary nutrient density. It boasts a staggering 92 of the 102 minerals that our bodies require. Among these, it's particularly high in iodine and selenium, both crucial for proper thyroid function. Moreover, it's an excellent source of vitamins like B2 and B9 (known as riboflavin and folate, respectively), amino acids, and antioxidants.

Regular consumption of Irish Sea Moss can result in improved digestion due to its high fiber content. Its gelatinous nature aids in soothing the mucous membrane throughout the body, notably in the respiratory system, making it a powerful tool against cold, flu, and more serious respiratory conditions.

Cultivation and Sourcing:

True to its name, Irish Sea Moss is ocean-farmed on the rocky shores, preferably in protected ocean areas to ensure that the seaweed can grow without being affected by environmental contaminants or pollutants. When sourcing, prioritize suppliers who can ensure the Sea Moss is wildcrafted, meaning it has been harvested directly from its natural habitat, thereby maintaining its nutrient density.

Preparation and Usage:

One of the most common forms to consume Irish Sea Moss is as a gel. To prepare, it should first be thoroughly washed and soaked for 12-24 hours. Then, it's boiled until soft, and finally, blended until it forms a smooth gel. This Sea Moss gel can be added to a variety of dishes, including smoothies, soups, desserts, and sauces. Additionally, it can be applied topically as a skin-soothing mask.

Dosage should start minimally, with just a teaspoon of Sea Moss gel a day, gradually increasing as the body becomes accustomed to it. While it's generally safe for most individuals, those with specific health conditions, particularly related to the thyroid, should consult a health practitioner before starting any new supplement regimen.

Storing and Preserving:

Freshly prepared Sea Moss gel can be stored in the refrigerator for up to three weeks. If stored in the freezer, it will maintain its potency for several months. Always use a clean, airtight container for storage to prevent contamination and premature spoilage.

In closing, Irish Sea Moss serves as a testament to the ocean's potent healing abilities. As we incorporate it into our diets, we embrace the wisdom of Dr. Sebi and his message of holistic health through nature's bounty.

Muicle: The Multifaceted Powerhouse

Muicle, scientifically named Justicia spicigera, holds a significant place in Dr. Sebi's array of approved herbs. Widely known across Central and South America, especially in Mexico, this potent herb has been an integral part of traditional medicine for centuries.

Health Benefits:

Muicle is cherished for its vast range of medicinal properties. Traditionally, it has been utilized for respiratory ailments, such as coughs, asthma, and bronchitis. The leaves of Muicle contain various bioactive compounds, including flavonoids and phenolics, which are thought to exert these therapeutic effects.

Furthermore, the plant is recognized for its potent antioxidant and anti-inflammatory properties, which can aid in battling various health conditions. It's also reputed to have blood-purifying qualities and has been used to alleviate gastrointestinal issues like diarrhea.

Cultivation and Sourcing:

Muicle is a perennial plant thriving in tropical climates. It grows optimally in well-drained soils under full sun exposure. In sourcing Muicle, it is crucial to ensure that it is organically grown, free of synthetic pesticides and fertilizers. The plant's quality can be verified through proper documentation, tracing back to its origin, cultivation methods, and harvesting process.

Preparation and Usage:

Muicle is commonly prepared as a tea or infusion, with its leaves steeped in hot water. The resulting brew is a deep red, indicative of its rich content of health-promoting compounds.

Storage and Preservation:

Maintaining the freshness and potency of Muicle requires proper storage. The dried leaves should be kept in an airtight container away from direct sunlight and moisture. This will keep the herb potent and effective for longer periods.

In summary, Muicle is a versatile herb with a wide array of health benefits. Its remarkable medicinal properties combined with its accessibility make it an excellent addition to the holistic health regimen. As you embrace the alkaline path, let Muicle be a robust ally in your quest for a vibrant, balanced, and thriving life. As always, remember that the key to deriving the most benefits from these powerful herbs lies in using them responsibly and under professional guidance.

Oregano: The Versatile Powerhouse

Oregano, botanically known as Origanum vulgare, is a commonly used herb in both culinary and medicinal applications. This perennial herb, found in Dr. Sebi's list of approved herbs, boasts a multitude of health benefits that make it a versatile addition to anyone's herbal repertoire.

Health Benefits:

Packed with antioxidants and antibacterial properties, oregano is widely known for its potent immune-boosting qualities. It can help protect the body from harmful pathogens and improve overall immune response. Some studies also suggest that oregano may aid in managing inflammation, contributing to its role in maintaining overall wellness.

The herb is also reputed for its respiratory support. The essential oil extracted from oregano is often used as a natural remedy for conditions like cough, asthma, and bronchitis.

Cultivation and Sourcing:

Oregano is native to the Mediterranean region but has been adapted to grow in various climates worldwide. For optimal quality, oregano should be sourced from a trusted, organic supplier that ensures the herb is grown without the use of pesticides or harmful chemicals.

Preparation and Usage:

In a culinary setting, oregano leaves, fresh or dried, are used to season a wide variety of dishes. Medicinally, oregano can be taken in several forms. It can be steeped into a herbal tea, ingested in capsule form, or used as an essential oil.

Dr. Sebi recommends starting with a lower dose and adjusting as necessary, always paying attention to your body's response to avoid potential side effects such as upset stomach or allergic reactions.

Storage and Preservation:

To maintain the potency of oregano, it should be stored properly. If you have fresh oregano, it's best to keep it in the refrigerator wrapped in a slightly damp paper towel. Dried oregano should be stored in a cool, dark, and dry place, such as a pantry or cupboard.

Oregano represents the fusion of culinary delight and medicinal potency, truly embodying the versatile power of herbs in promoting health and well-being. As you integrate oregano into your diet and wellness routine, you are embracing Dr. Sebi's vision of holistic health through the power of nature's gifts.

Prodigiosa: The Miraculous Herb

Prodigiosa (Brickellia grandiflora), commonly known as the prodigious or miraculous herb, is a valued part of Dr. Sebi's approved herbs list. This plant native to Mexico has a history steeped in traditional medicine and is prized for its range of health benefits.

Health Benefits:

In traditional medicine, Prodigiosa is renowned for its effectiveness in digestive health support. It is frequently used as a remedy for stomach ailments, such as gastritis, acid reflux, and indigestion. Additionally, it's believed to help manage blood sugar levels, which has made it a key player in natural treatments for diabetes.

Cultivation and Sourcing:

As a native plant to Mexico, Prodigiosa thrives in a warm, sunny climate. The sourcing of this herb should focus on its organic, wildcrafted variety, untouched by pesticides or chemical fertilizers. Suppliers should provide transparent information regarding the plant's origin and the farming practices employed.

Preparation and Usage:

Prodigiosa is commonly prepared as a tea, with the leaves steeped in hot water to extract their beneficial compounds. Due to its potent properties, the dosage of this herb must be carefully monitored. It is recommended to follow guidance from a naturopathic doctor to ensure safe and effective use.

Storage and Preservation:

Preserving Prodigiosa involves drying the leaves and storing them in a cool, dark, and dry environment. An airtight container is ideal for maintaining the herb's freshness and potency over time. Proper storage extends the shelf-life of the herb and ensures it remains effective for its intended use.

Quassia: The Potent Bitterwood

Quassia Amara, or simply Quassia, known for its extraordinarily bitter taste, is a powerful medicinal plant highlighted in Dr. Sebi's recommended list of herbs. Originating from the tropical regions of the Americas, this plant has been used for centuries for its notable health properties.

Health Benefits:

Quassia's health benefits are largely attributed to its strong anti-parasitic properties. Traditional medicine systems utilize it for combating various forms of internal parasites, enhancing digestive health, and promoting overall well-being. Further, it's known to stimulate appetite and enhance bile production, promoting a healthy and efficient digestive system.

Cultivation and Sourcing:

Quassia grows primarily in tropical climates and prefers well-drained, fertile soils. When sourcing Quassia, it is essential to look for suppliers committed to sustainable harvesting and cultivation practices. As always, the highest quality will be found in organic, wildcrafted Quassia, free from harmful chemicals and pollutants.

Preparation and Usage:

Due to its strong bitter taste, Quassia is typically prepared as a tea or infusion to aid digestion.

Storage and Preservation:

When properly dried and stored, Quassia can retain its medicinal properties for an extended period. Storing in a cool, dark, and dry location within an airtight container will help maintain its freshness and potency.

Red Clover: The Detoxification Dynamo

Red Clover (Trifolium pratense), a favorite of Dr. Sebi, is an amazing flowering plant known for its beautiful purplish-red color and myriad medicinal properties. Native to Europe, Western Asia, and Northwest Africa, Red Clover has found its way into various traditional medicine systems around the world.

Health Benefits:

Renowned for its detoxification properties, Red Clover is often employed to cleanse the blood and rid the body of toxins. It contains a rich array of nutrients, including vitamin C, calcium, and magnesium, and a wealth of isoflavones - plant compounds that mimic estrogen and have been linked to numerous health benefits. It has been known to support women's health, particularly in terms of menopause relief and balancing hormone levels.

Cultivation and Sourcing:

Red Clover grows in meadows and fields, demonstrating a liking for well-drained, clay soils. When sourcing, prioritize organic, wildcrafted Red Clover, which guarantees it hasn't been exposed to harmful pesticides or other chemicals. Ensure your supplier follows ethical and sustainable cultivation and harvesting practices to preserve the plant's natural environment.

Preparation and Usage:

Red Clover can be used in various ways, such as teas, tinctures, and capsules. It's essential to start with small doses and gradually increase as the body adjusts.

Storage and Preservation:

Properly dried Red Clover can maintain its potency for a long duration if stored correctly. Keep it in a cool, dry, and dark place within an airtight container to retain its freshness and efficacy.

Red Clover holds a unique spot in Dr. Sebi's list of beneficial herbs, being a powerful detoxifier and a well-rounded health supplement. Its application should be accompanied by responsible sourcing, proper preparation, and suitable dosage to maximize its potential in promoting holistic health and wellness.

Sarsaparilla: The Vibrant Vitality Booster

Sarsaparilla, also known scientifically as Smilax officinalis, is another herb greatly valued in Dr. Sebi's alkaline botanical repertoire. This chapter delves into the captivating world of Sarsaparilla, its health benefits, growth habits, sourcing guidelines, and usage recommendations.

Native to Central and South America, Sarsaparilla is a perennial vine that's been used for centuries due to its array of medicinal properties. The roots of this plant are particularly beneficial and are known for their unique flavor and potent health-boosting qualities.

Health Benefits:

Sarsaparilla is known for its detoxifying and purifying properties, making it an excellent aid for liver health. It helps cleanse the body of toxins, promoting overall health and wellbeing. The root is also packed with beneficial plant compounds, including saponins, which have antioxidant properties that protect your cells from damage.

Moreover, Sarsaparilla is used to balance hormones and boost vitality, and it's traditionally been used as a tonic for sexual health. It also aids in reducing inflammation, and it's been studied for its potential to alleviate symptoms related to psoriasis and other skin conditions.

Cultivation and Sourcing:

Sarsaparilla thrives in tropical and temperate climates with a preference for rich, well-drained soils. When sourcing Sarsaparilla, it is crucial to connect with suppliers who adhere to sustainable harvesting methods, given that the root is the most sought-after part of the plant.

Preparation and Usage:

The root of Sarsaparilla can be used in various ways. It can be boiled to create a beneficial tea or decoction, or it can be dried and powdered for encapsulation. As with any herb, it's advisable to start with small doses and adjust according to your body's response and tolerance.

Storage and Preservation:

Storing Sarsaparilla appropriately ensures it retains its beneficial properties. Keep it in a cool, dry, and dark place, preferably in an airtight container. If you have powdered Sarsaparilla, keep it away from direct light and heat to preserve its potency.

Sarsaparilla is a botanical gem from the heart of tropical forests, its vine symbolizing our continuous journey toward health and vitality. With its potent properties and extensive health benefits, it rightfully belongs in Dr. Sebi's approved herbs. As we incorporate Sarsaparilla into our health regimen, we imbibe a part of the forest's rich vitality and connect with our body's inherent potential for healing and rejuvenation.

Stinging Nettle: The Powerhouse Herb

Stinging Nettle, or scientifically known as Urtica dioica, holds a special place in Dr. Sebi's approved herbs for its array of health benefits. Rich in vital nutrients, this powerful herb is a force to be reckoned with when it comes to supporting overall well-being.

Health Benefits:

Stinging nettle is laden with beneficial compounds, making it a nutritional powerhouse. It is an excellent source of vitamins, including Vitamins A, C, K, as well as several B vitamins. Besides, it's also rich in minerals such as iron, magnesium, phosphorus, potassium, and calcium.

One of the most renowned benefits of stinging nettle is its ability to alleviate allergy symptoms. It acts as a natural antihistamine, helping to relieve sneezing, itching, and runny nose associated with allergic rhinitis.

Furthermore, stinging nettle can support urinary health. It has been used traditionally to alleviate symptoms of urinary tract infections and benign prostatic hyperplasia. It is also believed to support joint health, potentially reducing pain and inflammation associated with conditions such as arthritis.

Cultivation and Sourcing:

Stinging nettle is native to Europe, Asia, northern Africa, and western North America. It thrives in rich soil and prefers moist, shaded environments. If sourcing wild nettle, ensure that it is collected from unpolluted areas to avoid the potential accumulation of harmful substances.

If you prefer to buy instead of forage, ensure you find a trusted supplier who guarantees organically grown and sustainably harvested stinging nettle.

Preparation and Usage:
Stinging nettle can be consumed as a tea, cooked like spinach, or even made into a tincture. However, caution should be taken when handling fresh nettle due to its stinging hairs, hence its name. Cooking or drying neutralizes this effect, making it safe for consumption.

Storage and Preservation:
Fresh stinging nettle should be refrigerated and used within a few days for optimal freshness. For longer storage, stinging nettle can be dried and stored in a cool, dark, dry place in an airtight container. It can remain potent for up to a year if properly stored.

Incorporating stinging nettle into your herbal regimen can significantly enhance your health and well-being. Its diverse range of benefits makes it a versatile herb that aligns with Dr. Sebi's approach to holistic health.

Tila: The Soothing Nervine Herb

Tila, known scientifically as Tilia, is a genus of trees known in English as linden or lime trees. Tila flowers, endorsed by Dr. Sebi for their numerous health benefits, are harvested from these trees. Known for its soothing and calming properties, Tila is a go-to herb for stress relief and promoting tranquility.

Health Benefits:

One of the major benefits of Tila is its ability to reduce anxiety and induce relaxation. Its mild sedative effect has earned it a place in many sleep-aid tea blends. The herb also supports digestion and helps alleviate symptoms of indigestion such as bloating and gas. Moreover, it is known to help reduce inflammation, lower blood pressure, and alleviate symptoms of colds and coughs.

Cultivation and Sourcing:

Tilia trees are prevalent in temperate climates in the Northern Hemisphere. When sourcing Tila, it's important to focus on the quality of the flowers, which should ideally be organically grown and free from pesticides and other harmful chemicals.

Preparation and Usage:

Tila is traditionally prepared as a tea by steeping the dried flowers in boiling water for about 10 minutes. The taste is mild, often described as sweet and floral, making it a pleasant herb to consume regularly. Although the dosage can vary depending on the specific ailment being addressed, a common recommendation is to consume one to three cups of Tila tea per day.

Storage and Preservation:

Dried Tila flowers should be stored in a cool, dark place in an airtight container. This helps to maintain their potency and protect them from moisture, light, and pests.

Valerian Root: The Peaceful Sleep Promoter

Valerian (Valeriana officinalis), an herb beloved by Dr. Sebi, is a perennial flowering plant native to Europe and parts of Asia. The plant's root is commonly used in herbal medicine due to its myriad of health benefits, especially its potent effects on sleep and relaxation.

Health Benefits:

Valerian Root is most famous for its ability to promote a good night's sleep. It is used worldwide as a natural sleep aid, helping individuals fall asleep faster and improve sleep quality. Additionally, its calming properties make it useful in managing anxiety and stress. Studies also indicate its potential in easing menstrual and stomach cramps.

Cultivation and Sourcing:

Valerian is relatively easy to grow, thriving best in locations with full sun or partial shade and moist, well-draining soil. When sourcing Valerian Root, it is vital to ensure it is free from pesticides, chemical fertilizers, and other potential toxins. Prioritize suppliers who follow organic farming practices to maintain the herb's integrity and maximize its therapeutic benefits.

Preparation and Usage:

Valerian Root is commonly consumed as a tea or in capsule form. As a tea, it offers a slightly bitter taste, which can be enhanced with sweeteners or other herbs. When it comes to dosage, it's recommended to follow the instructions on the product packaging or consult with a healthcare professional.

Storage and Preservation:

Valerian Root, particularly when dried, should be stored in a cool, dark place, ideally in a well-sealed container to protect it from moisture, light, and pests. Proper storage ensures the preservation of its active compounds and longevity of use.

Valerian Root is a remarkable herb that carries significant benefits, particularly for those struggling with sleep issues or seeking to manage stress. As with all herbs in Dr. Sebi's approved list, understanding its properties, correct usage, and storage is key to reaping its full benefits.

Yellow Dock: The Bountiful Blood Purifier

Yellow Dock (Rumex crispus), a standout herb in Dr. Sebi's list, is a perennial flowering plant native to Europe and Western Asia but now found worldwide. Its yellow root, from which it gets its name, is the primary part used in herbal medicine.

Health Benefits:

Yellow Dock is traditionally renowned for its exceptional blood-purifying properties. It assists in toxin removal and enhances overall blood quality, leading to numerous health benefits. Rich in iron, it's often used to treat anemia and boost red blood cell production. Its antioxidant properties protect cells from oxidative damage, while its anti-inflammatory effects help manage various inflammation-related conditions.

Cultivation and Sourcing:

Yellow Dock is a versatile plant that thrives in many environments, often seen in fields, roadsides, and waste grounds. When sourcing Yellow Dock, seek out suppliers that adhere to sustainable and organic practices, avoiding herbs exposed to pesticides or other chemical contaminants.

Preparation and Usage:

Yellow Dock root can be prepared in a variety of forms. As a tea, it's a warming, nourishing drink. It can also be tinctured or encapsulated for ease of use. The dosage should be individualized according to specific health needs and goals, always starting small and adjusting as necessary.

Storage and Preservation:

Dried Yellow Dock root should be stored in a cool, dark, and dry environment, ideally in an airtight container to preserve its potency and prevent moisture damage.

These herbs provide the basis for the cleansing teas, infusions, and decoctions you'll learn to prepare in the following chapters. Each has its own unique properties that can aid in your journey towards full-body detox and lifelong health.

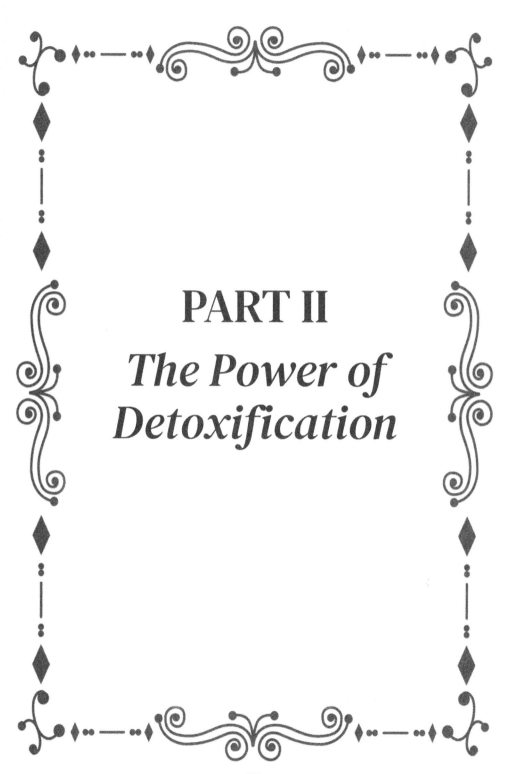

PART II
The Power of Detoxification

The Role of Alkaline Herbs In The Detoxification Process

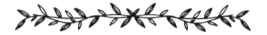

Alkaline herbs play a pivotal role in the detoxification process. These specific herbs, recommended by Dr. Sebi, are crucial for helping the body eliminate toxins and naturally restore our internal balance. These potent botanicals have a combination of properties that make them perfect for detoxification protocols.

The alkaline advantage

Alkaline herbs, as their name implies, have an alkaline feature that rectifies the effects acidity may provoke within our body. Indeed, high acidity levels can lead to health problems, from discomforts like heartburn to more severe conditions like acidosis. By incorporating alkaline herbs into your diet, you can maintain a balanced pH level and create an environment that promotes overall health and wellness.

Supporting the well-being of organs

Every alkaline herb possesses qualities that assist our organs. For instance, herbs like dandelion and burdock optimize liver functioning. They also eliminate toxins from the bloodstream and stimulate bile production, a substance that aids in fat digestion and absorption of fat-soluble vitamins.

Strengthening the immune system and digestive health

Many alkaline herbs are renowned for bolstering our immune system. For instance, due to its immune-boosting properties, elderberry has traditionally been employed to fight flu and colds. By improving the immune system's effectiveness, alkaline herbs assist our body in resisting and recovering from illnesses. Several herbs with alkaline properties also boost the digestive system's functioning by assisting our body in the smooth breakdown of foods, absorption of essential nutrients, and expulsion of waste. Sarsaparilla, for instance, is renowned for its ability to address ailments, improving our digestive wellness.

Antioxidant and anti-inflammatory properties

Chronic diseases are often caused by inflammation and oxidative stress. Alkaline herbs have been found to have inflammatory and antioxidant properties, which can help counteract these factors contributing to the arising of such diseases. For example, herbs like bladder wrack and sea moss are known for their abundance of antioxidants through which they can effectively fight radicals. Additionally, herbs like blue vervain contain natural compounds designed to fight inflammation.

To summarize, herbs with alkaline properties facilitate the body's natural detoxification pathways by boosting our immune system, maintaining a balanced pH level, and supporting our organs' well-being. Moving forward to the next chapter, we will further explore an in-depth guide on performing a thorough body detox using these potent plants.

A Step-By-Step Guide for A Full-Body Detox

Embarking on a full-body detox journey can often feel very overwhelming. Nevertheless, you can turn this journey into a feasible and fulfilling experience by taking a systematic and organized approach. Here we prepared a comprehensive breakdown of all the steps involved in a full-body detox experience, emphasizing the relevance of incorporating alkaline herbs throughout each phase.

Step 1: the preparation

It is essential to pay attention to the preparation phase when it comes to the detoxification process. First and foremost, you should eliminate alcohol, processed foods, caffeine, and sugars from your diet. Contrarily, it would help to concentrate on consuming whole, plant-based foods. During this stage, it is incredibly beneficial for your organism to introduce alkaline herbs within your daily routine. Getting into the habit of drinking tea containing herbs, for instance, elderberry (sambucus nigra) or sarsaparilla (smilax ornata), can support you in preparing your body for the detoxification process.

Step 2: the cleansing phase

During this phase, increasing your intake of alkaline herbs is vital. The main goal is cleansing your colon, purifying your blood, and supporting the optimal functioning of organs, like the liver and kidneys, that play a vital role in detoxification. Enjoy some tea infused with burdock root (Arctium lappa) and dandelion (Taraxacum officinale), as they stimulate your bile production, support your liver health, and eliminate toxins from your bloodstream. Additionally, you can incorporate herbs such as cascara Sagrada (Rhamnus purshiana) to purify your colon and stimulate regular bowel movements.

Step 3: the rebuilding phase:

After detoxification, the body enters third phase, known as "rebuilding phase".

During this stage, the focus is placed on restoring the body's processes, boosting immunity, and enhancing well-being. To support this stage of the detoxifying process, including sea moss (Chondrus crispus) and bladder wrack (Fucus vesiculosus) in your diet is beneficial. These herbs are known for their high levels of minerals and revitalizing properties, which can help your body replenish nutrients and restore an overall balance.

Step 4: the maintenance phase

In this final step, known as the "maintenance phase," the objective is to uphold the habits you developed during detoxification and maintain the body's newfound equilibrium. Incorporating alkaline herbs into your daily food consumption is essential, making relevant adjustments based on your body's requirements and reactions.

Remember that detoxification is a consistent process, not a one-time occurrence.

It can be supported by consuming alkaline herbs and maintaining a balanced and mindful lifestyle.

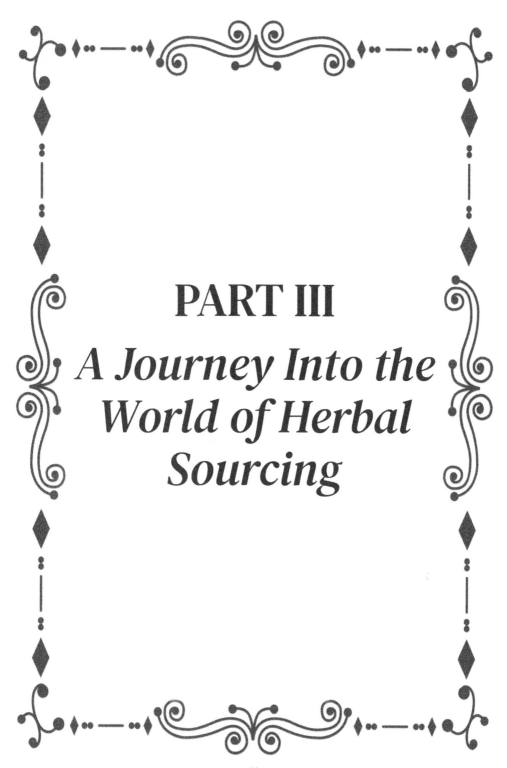

PART III

A Journey Into the World of Herbal Sourcing

Recognizing the Importance of Quality in the Practice of Herbal Sourcing

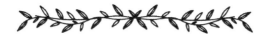

Dr. Sebi's alkaline healing philosophy emphasizes the importance of high-quality herbs.

Indeed, the success of any herbal regimen relies on the purity and strength of the herbs employed. When sourcing herbs, quality is influenced by several factors, such as harvesting methods, growing conditions, processing techniques, and storage. Awareness of the relevance of each of these aspects can help you make more educated choices when sourcing your herbs.

Factors to keep in mind when sourcing Dr. Sebi's medicinal herbs

When sourcing Dr. Sebi's medical herbs, it goes far beyond locating a supplier and making a purchase. It involves having elevated judgment skills and understanding. To ensure the authenticity and integrity of your herbs, you need to consider several factors, such as:

Cultivation versus wildcrafting: when it comes to herbs, there are two methods to obtain them. Wildcrafted herbs are harvested from natural habitats, while cultivated herbs are grown in controlled environments. Both approaches have advantages and disadvantages, which we will explore in the following sections.

Organic certification: it guarantees that the herbs have been cultivated without the use of synthetic pesticides and fertilizers, contributing to your well-being, as well as to the well-being of our planet.

Effectiveness and freshness: the quality and effectiveness of herbs can diminish over time or due to poor storage conditions. Being able to recognize these factors will assist you in avoiding low-quality or sour herbs.

Ethically sourced products: when sourcing herbs, prioritizing sustainability and ethical practices is crucial. Being aware of the origins and methods of herb sourcing can help guarantee that your quest for healing also contributes to our planet's and communities' well-being.

You will gain the essential knowledge to navigate the realm of herbal sourcing confidently through this book. Our goal is to assist you throughout your journey toward health by ensuring you obtain the highest quality herbs to meet your specific needs.

PART IV

Sourcing Guidelines for Dr. Sebi's Medical Herbs

Exploring the Concept of Wildcrafted Herbs

When gathering herbs, it is vital to understand the idea of wildcrafting. Wildcrafting is harvesting plants from their natural environment for culinary, medical, or other purposes. This approach suggests that the plant has thrived in its habitat and retains its potential in terms of healing properties, as it has grown free from human contamination. Wildcrafted herbs are precious because they are thought to have elevated effectiveness and therapeutic benefits.

Dr. Sebi's medical herbs are often gathered from their native habitats, which makes them wildcrafted. These herbs grow naturally and absorb nutrients from their surroundings, allowing them to adapt to the climate and fend off pests and diseases. As a result, these plants often develop into resilient specimens with a concentration of beneficial compounds.

However, it is crucial to acknowledge that wildcrafting should be approached with caution and sustainable practices to prevent excessive depletion of natural plant populations. Reputable herbal suppliers will provide you with in-depth details regarding their wildcrafting techniques, ensuring they are environmentally conscious.

Delving into wildcrafted herbs, you will develop a sense of appreciation and understanding of their purity and power. This awareness you will grow will also help you to appreciate the overall concept of ethical sourcing. In the following sections of this book, we will thoroughly explore the aspects worthy of considering when sourcing wildcrafted herbs. Likewise, we will also further discuss strategies you can employ to establish whether your herbs have been harvested responsibly.

The Relevance of Organic Herbs

When it comes to sourcing Dr. Sebi's herbs, it is crucial to prioritize our choices. Organic farming places an emphasis on preserving people's health and the ecosystem. Accordingly, organic herbs are cultivated without the employment of bioengineered genes (GMOs), sewage sludge-based or petroleum-based fertilizers, or synthetic pesticides. These substances can cause harmful impacts not just on the plants themselves but also on the water, local wildlife, soil, air, and ultimately our well-being.

When herbs are grown organically, they are allowed to grow at their natural pace, under natural conditions. This method of farming preserves the natural vitality of the herbs and ensures that they are free from potentially harmful residues. Organic certification guarantees that the herbs were grown, harvested, stored, processed, and packaged according to rigorous standards. It also guarantees that the herbs were not fumigated or irradiated during storage and packaging, processes that can diminish the therapeutic qualities of the herbs.

Therefore, it's important to purchase organic herbs whenever possible. Not only does this promote better health for you, but it also supports sustainable farming practices and contributes to the health of the planet. In the next sections, we will go over how to identify high-quality herbal products and the impact of the growing environment on herb quality.

Identifying High-Quality Herbal Products

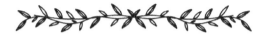

Once you've gained an understanding of wildcrafted and organic herbs, the next critical step is identifying high-quality herbal products. The market is flooded with numerous herbal products, but not all of them meet the standards for quality and effectiveness.

High-quality herbs share several defining characteristics. The first characteristic is vibrant color. Herbs should have bright, saturated colors, indicative of a high concentration of the vital life force and nutrients. Dull or overly dry herbs may not provide the full range of therapeutic benefits.

The second characteristic is aroma. High-quality herbs should have a strong, characteristic aroma, signaling the presence of volatile oils and other aromatic compounds, which are often the active ingredients in medicinal herbs.

Thirdly, the texture and integrity of the herbs are also essential. The herbs should be intact and not overly fragmented. For dried herbs, they should still retain some degree of suppleness and not crumble too easily.

The fourth characteristic is the taste. Although not always pleasant, the taste of herbs can also indicate their quality. High-quality herbs often have a potent flavor profile, another indicator of the concentration of active compounds.

Packaging is another significant factor in maintaining herbal quality. Look for products packaged in dark glass or other materials that protect the herbs from light and moisture, which can degrade the herbs over time.

Finally, a company's reputation is also crucial. Do your research and choose companies known for their commitment to quality, transparency, and ethical sourcing. Consider if the company provides clear and detailed information about the source of their herbs, their farming practices, and their processing methods.

Remember, the effectiveness of Dr. Sebi's herbal remedies is directly linked to the quality of the herbs used. Therefore, it's vital to source the best quality products to ensure optimal health benefits.

The Impact of the Growing Environment on Herb Quality

The environment in which an herb grows plays a crucial role in determining its quality and medicinal value. Herbs are deeply influenced by the conditions of their growing environment, which can significantly impact the concentrations of beneficial compounds they contain. This section will delve into the impact of the growing environment on herb quality and why it is important to take it into account when sourcing Dr. Sebi's medical herbs.

Firstly, the soil quality is of utmost importance. Nutrient-rich soil, free from contaminants and heavy metals, produces herbs with high nutrient content. In contrast, herbs grown in poor quality soil or soil contaminated with pesticides and other chemicals might not only lack the necessary nutrients but may also carry harmful substances. This is one of the reasons why wildcrafted and organic herbs are often more potent and safer; they grow in pristine, fertile soil in their natural habitats, where they can absorb a wide range of nutrients.

Secondly, the climate and weather conditions can significantly affect the growth of the herbs and the concentration of their active compounds. For example, certain herbs grow better in warm, tropical climates, while others thrive in cooler, temperate zones. The amounts of sunlight, rainfall, and temperature fluctuations can all influence the development of the herbs and their biochemical composition.

The biodiversity of the growing area also impacts the quality of the herbs. Herbs grown in biodiverse environments, surrounded by various other plants and animals, are generally healthier and more potent. This biodiversity can contribute to the robustness of the plants, helping them develop a rich array of compounds to adapt to their environment.

Lastly, the timing of the harvest also plays a crucial role. Each herb has a specific harvesting time when its active compounds are at their peak. Harvesting at the wrong time can lead to a significant decrease in the potency of the herbs.

By understanding the role of the growing environment, you can make informed decisions when sourcing Dr. Sebi's medical herbs. Always strive to choose herbs that are grown in their indigenous environments under optimal conditions, and harvested at the right time, to ensure you are getting the highest quality and most beneficial herbs.

PART V
The Process of Sourcing Medical Herbs

Research: Understanding the Plant's Natural Habitat

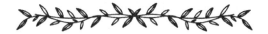

D r. Sebi's medicinal herbs vary significantly in terms of their natural habitats, reflecting their unique adaptations and growth requirements. To ensure that you're sourcing the highest quality herbs, it's essential to understand these diverse habitats. The following sections provide in-depth information about the natural habitats of some key herbs recommended by Dr. Sebi.

Burdock Root (Arctium lappa): This plant is native to Europe and North Asia but has also been naturalized in parts of North America. It thrives in sunny locations with well-draining soil. The plant prefers neutral to slightly alkaline pH levels. It can grow in a variety of soil types but particularly favors nitrogen-rich soil. When sourcing Burdock root, check if the supplier's growing conditions mimic these preferences.

Sea Moss (Chondrus crispus): As its name suggests, Sea Moss, also known as Irish Moss, thrives in the ocean. It is native to the Atlantic coasts of Europe and North America. When sourcing Sea Moss, look for suppliers who harvest it from clean, unpolluted waters, preferably during spring, when its nutritional content is highest.

Sarsaparilla (Smilax spp.): Sarsaparilla plants are native to tropical regions in the Americas and the Caribbean. They grow best in well-draining soil, under partial shade to full sun conditions. If the Sarsaparilla you are sourcing comes from areas mimicking these conditions, it is likely of high quality.

Elderberry (Sambucus nigra): Elderberries are native to Europe, Africa, and parts of Asia but have also been naturalized in the United States. These plants prefer sunny to partially shaded locations and can grow in various soil types, though they prefer moist, fertile soils.

Dandelion (Taraxacum officinale): Dandelion, native to Europe and Asia, is a hardy plant that can grow in a wide range of conditions. It prefers full sun to partial shade and well-drained soils. It can thrive in a broad spectrum of soil types and pH levels.

Bladderwrack (Fucus vesiculosus): Like Sea Moss, Bladderwrack is a type of seaweed. It is native to the North Sea coasts, the western Baltic Sea, and the Atlantic and Pacific Oceans. Look for Bladderwrack harvested from clean waters to ensure its quality.

Yellow Dock (Rumex crispus): This perennial herb is native to Europe and Western Asia but has naturalized in many parts of North America. Yellow Dock thrives in full sun to partial shade conditions, prefers slightly acidic to neutral pH, and can tolerate a wide range of soil types, including heavy clay.

Stinging Nettle (Urtica dioica): Stinging Nettle is a hardy plant that grows in temperate regions worldwide. It prefers rich, moist soil with a neutral to slightly alkaline pH and can tolerate partial shade to full sun exposure.

Red Clover (Trifolium pratense): Red Clover is native to Europe, Western Asia, and northwest Africa, but it has been naturalized in many other regions. It thrives in loamy soil, prefers neutral to slightly alkaline pH, and needs full sun to partial shade.

Cascara Sagrada (Rhamnus purshiana): This plant is native to western North America, from northern California to British Columbia. It thrives in moist, acidic soils, and prefers shady or partially shady environments.

Chaparral (Larrea tridentata): Chaparral is native to the deserts of southwestern North America, from southern California to west Texas and northern Mexico. It thrives in arid conditions, in sandy or rocky soils, under full sun exposure.

Understanding the natural habitats of these herbs can provide you with valuable information about the conditions they need to grow effectively. This knowledge will help you ensure that the herbs you're sourcing are of the highest possible quality.

Remember that these are just a few of the numerous medicinal herbs recommended by Dr. Sebi. Each plant has its unique habitat preferences, which can significantly impact its growth and medicinal properties. Therefore, taking the time to research these habitats and ensuring your suppliers adhere to them can make a significant difference in the quality of the herbs you source.

Inspection: How to Assess the Quality of Herbs

As we continue our journey to source high-quality medicinal herbs, it is paramount to understand the inspection process and the key indicators that point towards a high-quality product. While you might not always be able to physically inspect the herbs, knowing what to look for will guide your purchase decisions.

1. Visual Inspection:

A primary and straightforward method to assess the quality of herbs is visual inspection. The color of the herb can be a significant indicator of its freshness and quality. Herbs should typically retain the vibrant color they possess in their natural state. Any discoloration might be a sign of poor storage conditions, age, or improper drying methods.

Consider the example of Burdock root (Arctium lappa), a herb favored by Dr. Sebi. When freshly dried, it should maintain a light brown or tan color. If the color appears dull or overly darkened, it could indicate that the herb has aged significantly or has been exposed to unfavorable conditions.

2. Olfactory Inspection:

Smell is another powerful tool for assessing herbal quality. Herbs should emit a fresh and characteristic aroma. If the smell is faint, uncharacteristic, or unpleasant, it could indicate spoilage, age, or contamination. For instance, Oregano (Origanum vulgare) should have a fresh, somewhat strong, and penetrating smell. A lack of aroma or an off smell may signal a compromised product.

3. Tactile Inspection:

Feel the herbs, if possible. They should retain some resilience. Brittle herbs might suggest that they were over-dried, potentially losing their potency in the process. However, certain herbs, like Sea Moss (Chondrus crispus), are an exception to this rule as they naturally dry to a crispy texture.

4. Purchase from Reputable Sources:

While all the above points help, the best guarantee of quality is to purchase from a reputable source. A trustworthy supplier will have transparent sourcing practices, fair trade certifications, organic certifications, or other verifiable quality standards.

5. Certificate of Analysis:

A Certificate of Analysis (CoA) is a document issued by Quality Assurance that confirms a regulated product meets its product specification. It contains the actual results obtained from testing performed as part of quality control of an individual batch of a product.

In the context of herbs, a CoA may include tests for identity (botanical or otherwise), purity, strength, and composition. It might also provide results for any potential contaminants, like heavy metals or pesticides.

Requesting and reviewing the CoA can provide peace of mind regarding the quality and safety of the herbs.

Remember, sourcing high-quality herbs is a crucial aspect of embracing the alkaline herbal path that Dr. Sebi advocated. Being informed and vigilant about the quality of your herbs will ensure that you're receiving the maximum health benefits these plants offer.

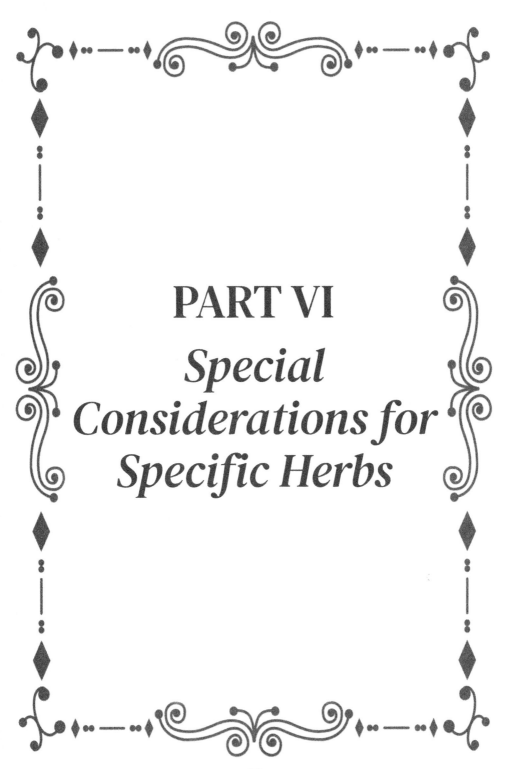

PART VI
Special Considerations for Specific Herbs

Unique Sourcing Considerations for Specific Herbs

While the general guidelines for sourcing herbs apply across the board, it's important to note that certain herbs require special considerations due to their unique characteristics. Here, we will explore a few such herbs, particularly those endorsed by Dr. Sebi, and discuss their specific sourcing considerations.

1. Irish Sea Moss (Chondrus crispus):

Irish Sea Moss, a type of red algae that grows in the cool Atlantic waters, has unique sourcing considerations due to its marine origin. When sourcing sea moss, ensure that it is wildcrafted – harvested directly from its natural oceanic environment. This ensures that the sea moss has absorbed a rich array of nutrients from its habitat, making it more beneficial to your health.

Avoid pool-grown sea moss, which often has a uniform color and lacks the natural taste and texture of wildcrafted sea moss. Pool-grown sea moss may also have fewer nutrients due to controlled growing conditions.

2. Sarsaparilla (Smilax ornata):

Sarsaparilla, native to South America, thrives in warm climates and is known for its medicinal root. It's crucial to source from suppliers who harvest the root responsibly, ensuring the plant's sustainability. When harvested correctly, the plant can regrow, providing a continuous source of this beneficial herb.

3. Stinging Nettle (Urtica dioica):

Stinging Nettle is native to Europe, Asia, North America, and Northern Africa. It grows best in nitrogen-rich soil, near stream banks, and on the edges of meadows. One unique sourcing consideration for Stinging Nettle is the handling of the plant itself. The leaves and stems have tiny hairs that can sting upon touch. Therefore, the plant must be handled carefully during harvest and processing.

Knowing the unique sourcing considerations of each herb not only allows you to ensure the quality of the product but also contributes to the preservation of these valuable plant species. Making an informed choice helps promote ethical and sustainable sourcing practices in the industry.

Seasonality and Harvesting Times for Key Herbs

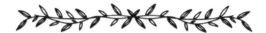

Understanding the best times to harvest herbs can greatly impact their potency and effectiveness. Similar to fruits and vegetables, herbs have specific times during the year when they are at their peak. Here, we will explore the optimal seasonality and harvesting times for some of Dr. Sebi's key herbs.

1. Burdock Root (Arctium lappa):

Burdock is a biennial plant, and the best time to harvest the root is during the fall of its first year or the spring of the second year. During these periods, the plant has stored up high levels of nutrients in the root, making it an optimal time for harvest.

2. Yellow Dock (Rumex crispus):

Yellow Dock, like Burdock, is a biennial plant. The roots are best harvested in late fall through early spring, when the plant's energy is stored in the root system. The leaves, however, can be harvested in the spring and early summer, when they are young and tender.

3. Dandelion (Taraxacum officinale):

Dandelion, a perennial plant, can be harvested almost year-round. However, the roots are best harvested in the fall when they are full of stored nutrients. The leaves are best when picked in the early spring when they are less bitter.

4. Elderberry (Sambucus nigra):

Elderberries are harvested in the late summer and early fall. The ripe, dark berries are collected for medicinal use, while the rest of the plant is generally avoided due to potential toxicity.

5. Sea Moss (Chondrus crispus):

Sea Moss, or Irish Moss, is typically harvested during the spring and summer months when it grows abundantly. Harvesting involves pulling the plant from the sea floor, ensuring a piece is left for regeneration.

6. Sarsaparilla (Smilax ornata):

Sarsaparilla root is harvested in the autumn, once the plant's leaves have wilted and its energy has been transferred to the root.

7. Bladderwrack (Fucus vesiculosus):

Like Sea Moss, Bladderwrack is harvested from the sea. The best time for harvesting Bladderwrack is during the late spring and early summer when the plant is in its growth phase and rich in nutrients.

8. Stinging Nettle (Urtica dioica):

The leaves of the Stinging Nettle plant are harvested in the spring and can be used fresh or dried for later use. The roots, however, are harvested in the autumn.

Always keep these harvesting times in mind when purchasing your herbs, as they greatly affect the potency and healing properties of each plant. It's a good practice to communicate with your supplier and ask about their harvesting practices to ensure they align with these ideal timeframes.

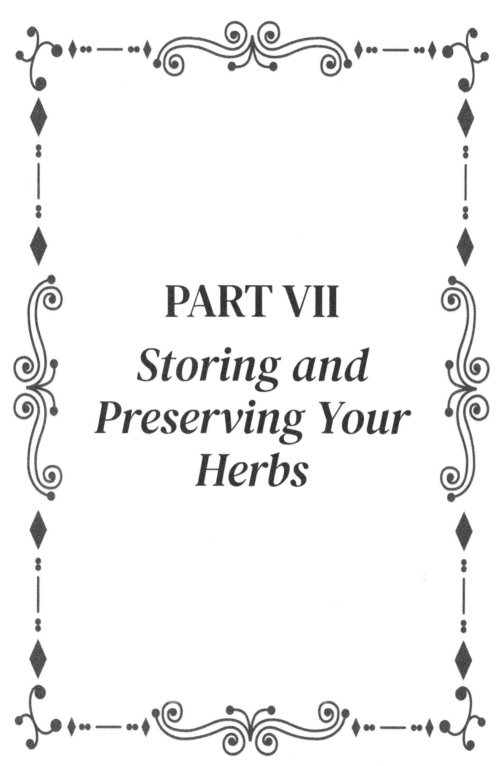

PART VII
Storing and Preserving Your Herbs

Proper Storage to Maintain Potency and Freshness

The journey to ensure the highest quality of Dr. Sebi's approved alkaline herbs doesn't stop at sourcing; it extends into how we store these herbs. Proper storage is as essential as careful selection to maintain the potency, freshness, and healing properties of the herbs. Controlling the temperature is a crucial aspect of this process. Herbs need to be stored in a cool place, as excessive heat can degrade the active compounds in them, reducing their effectiveness. A temperature-controlled pantry or a cabinet away from heat sources like the oven or stove is often the best location to store your herbs. Alongside this, it's also important to shield them from light. Direct exposure to sunlight should be avoided, as UV rays can gradually degrade the quality of the herbs over time, compromising their efficacy and freshness.

Delving deeper into storage practices, it's important to understand that each herb comes with its unique requirements, but certain general principles often apply. Moisture is the enemy of most dried herbs; it can lead to mold growth and degradation of the herb's quality. So, keeping your herbs in a dry environment is crucial. Packaging also plays a significant role in maintaining an herb's potency. Glass containers are generally preferred over plastic ones because they don't leach any chemicals into the herbs, maintaining their purity.

Also, remember to store herbs in airtight containers. Exposure to air can make herbs stale, and they might lose their flavor and healing properties. Moreover, it's good practice to keep your herbs away from strong-smelling foods or spices, as they can absorb odors, which may interfere with their natural aroma.

It's important to note that proper storage isn't just about preserving the herbs' therapeutic properties. It also ensures you're getting the most out of your investment in these potent healers, by prolonging their shelf life. Lastly, always label your herbs with the name and the date of purchase. This practice helps keep track of freshness, ensuring you're always using herbs at their prime.

Preserving Herbs: Drying, Freezing, Infusing and Other Methods

Now let's turn our attention to the methods of preserving herbs. Preserving herbs allows you to maintain their potency over time, providing you with a ready supply of high-quality materials for your herbal remedies.

Drying is one of the most common and straightforward methods of preserving herbs. This method involves removing the moisture from the herbs to prevent decay and preserve their therapeutic properties. Depending on the herb, you might want to air dry, use a dehydrator, or even an oven at the lowest temperature. Remember, you want to keep the temperature low to preserve as many beneficial compounds as possible.

Freezing herbs is another method of preservation. This is particularly suitable for herbs that don't dry well or lose their potency when dried. To freeze herbs, you can simply place them in freezer-safe bags or containers. Some herbs can also be frozen in ice cube trays with a bit of water, providing convenient, pre-measured amounts ready for use in your recipes.

Infusing involves steeping herbs in a substance, such as oil, vinegar, or alcohol, to extract their beneficial properties. The resulting infusions can then be used in a variety of applications, from cooking to skincare to medicinal remedies. Infusing allows you to create potent herbal products that can be stored for extended periods, providing you with a ready supply of your favorite remedies.

Tincturing: This is a process of soaking herbs in alcohol to extract the active compounds. The alcohol acts as a preservative, allowing the tincture to be stored for a long time without losing its potency. Tinctures are typically taken in small doses, either directly or diluted in water or juice.

Making Herbal Salts and Sugars: Herbs can be blended with salt or sugar, creating a unique and flavorful addition to cooking and baking. These mixtures can be stored in airtight containers and used as desired.

Canning: Herbs can also be preserved through canning. Herbs are packed into canning jars along with a preservation medium such as vinegar, oil, or a sugar syrup, then the jars are sealed and heated to kill off any bacteria, yeasts, or molds that might cause the herbs to spoil.

Honey Infusion: Herbs can be infused in honey, which not only preserves their medicinal qualities but also adds a sweet flavor, making the remedy more enjoyable to take.

Making Herbal Vinegars: Herbs are steeped in vinegar to create a flavorful addition to salads, marinades, and other dishes. The acidity of the vinegar acts as a natural preservative.

Capsulizing: For those who find the taste of certain herbs unpalatable, capsulizing can be an excellent method. The dried herbs are ground into a fine powder and then filled into capsules. This also allows for precise dosage control.

These additional methods provide you with a range of options for preserving the medicinal properties of your herbs, enabling you to choose the method that best suits your personal preferences and the specific properties of each herb. Remember, the goal of preservation is to maintain the quality and potency of the herbs, so it's important to handle them gently and store them correctly after preservation.

PART VIII
Grinding Dr. Sebi's Herbs

Grinding Dr. Sebi's Herbs: Why Grinding Is Necessary

Herbs come to us in many forms but grinding them into a more manageable state is often the first step in incorporating them into a healing routine. Grinding Dr. Sebi's herbs serves several important purposes, and understanding why this process is necessary is essential for optimal use of these potent plants.

Firstly, grinding herbs increases their surface area, enabling the active compounds in the plants to be released more effectively. This makes the resulting powder more potent, ensuring that you get the most out of every herb in your regime.

Secondly, ground herbs are more easily absorbed by the body. When herbs are finely ground, it's easier for your digestive system to break them down and absorb the beneficial compounds they contain. This ensures maximum absorption and use of the beneficial compounds in each herb.

Lastly, grinding herbs allows for easier and more consistent dosing. Because ground herbs are more uniform, it's simpler to measure an exact dose. This is particularly important when using medicinal herbs, as getting the right dose can be the key to achieving the desired effect.

In summary, grinding is a simple but essential step in preparing Dr. Sebi's herbs. It enhances potency, promotes absorption, and simplifies dosing, helping you get the most out of each plant's healing properties.

How To Grind Herbs Properly: Maximizing Efficiency and Potency

The process of grinding herbs is not merely a mechanical process, but an essential step in preserving the potency and bioavailability of the valuable compounds within them. For most of Dr. Sebi's recommended herbs, a quality grinder or a mortar and pestle will be needed to break the plant material down to the desired consistency.

Bear in mind, grinding generates heat, which can potentially degrade the delicate bioactive compounds in the herbs. This means it's crucial to take care during this process. Ideally, the herbs should be ground slowly and in small quantities to minimize heat production.

Moreover, the size of the grind matters as well. For example, a coarse grind may be ideal for making a decoction or an infusion, while a finer grind would be preferable when looking to encapsulate the herb or if it will be used as a component in topical applications.

Always ensure that your grinding equipment is clean and dry before use and try to process your herbs soon after grinding them. This helps to maintain their freshness and potency, maximizing their therapeutic potential. It is also good practice to clean your equipment thoroughly after each use to prevent cross-contamination between different herbs.

By learning how to grind your herbs correctly, you can ensure you're getting the most from Dr. Sebi's herbal recommendations, contributing to your journey towards optimal health.

To grind herbs effectively, you have several options depending on the herbs you're using and your personal preference. Here are some tools that you can consider:

Mortar and Pestle: This is the most traditional method for grinding herbs and is still widely used today. It's especially good for smaller quantities of herbs and allows for great control over the fineness of the grind. However, it can require a bit of effort and time, particularly for tougher, woody herbs.

Herb or Coffee Grinder: Electric or manual grinders can be very effective and save a lot of time and effort. They're great for grinding larger quantities of herbs quickly. However, they can generate more heat due to the speed of the grinding process, which can potentially degrade some of the delicate compounds in the herbs. Always aim to pulse rather than continuously grind to minimize this issue.

Spice Mill: A spice mill works similarly to a coffee grinder but is generally better at achieving a fine grind. They are a good choice for herbs that you want to be ground into a very fine powder.

Blender or Food Processor: These can work well for grinding large quantities of herbs, but they may not achieve as fine a grind as a spice mill or grinder.

No matter what tool you use, remember to clean it thoroughly before and after each use to avoid cross-contamination. Also, consider dedicating a specific grinder for your herbs if you're also using these tools for coffee or other foods to prevent mixing of flavors and scents.

Best Practices for Storing Ground Herbs

Once you've ground your herbs, it's paramount to store them correctly to ensure their potency, freshness, and medicinal properties are preserved. The foremost rule is to choose the right container. Airtight containers safeguard the herbs from air exposure, which can accelerate the degradation process. Glass jars with airtight lids are an excellent choice as they do not react with the herbs and are easy to sterilize. Ensure your jars are clean and completely dry before adding your herbs to prevent any moisture, which could lead to mold development.

When selecting a storage location, it's critical to consider the conditions. Light, heat, and moisture can quickly degrade your herbs, causing them to lose their potency. Therefore, choose a dark, cool, and dry place for storage. A cupboard away from heat sources such as the oven or stove is ideal. Also, avoid storing them in a location that experiences significant temperature fluctuations, like above a refrigerator.

The freshness of your herbs also relies on regular checkups. Make a habit of inspecting your stored herbs regularly. Look for signs of moisture or insect infestation. If you notice a change in the color, smell, or texture, it could mean that the herbs have started to lose their potency and it might be time to replace them.

Finally, remember that ground herbs generally have a shorter shelf life than whole herbs due to their increased surface area. Aim to grind only as much as you'll use within a few months to ensure maximum potency and freshness. And always label your containers with the date of grinding to help keep track of their freshness.

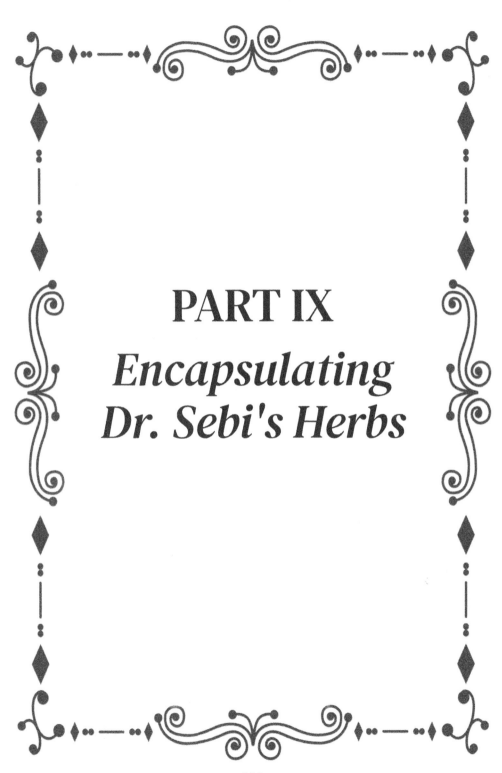

PART IX
Encapsulating Dr. Sebi's Herbs

Encapsulation Process

Encapsulation is a popular method to consume herbs, especially those that may have a somewhat bitter or unpleasant taste. This process involves filling small, digestible capsules with the ground herbs of your choice, creating a pill-like product that's easy to swallow and digest.

There are several benefits to encapsulating Dr. Sebi's herbs. First and foremost, it significantly enhances the ease of consumption. Many medicinal herbs, while potent in their effects, don't necessarily have the most pleasing flavors. Encapsulating these herbs can mask the taste while ensuring you receive their full benefits.

Secondly, encapsulation can aid in precision of dosage. Each capsule you create can contain a set amount of herbs, which simplifies knowing exactly how much you're consuming. This is especially beneficial if you're following a specific regimen that requires accurate dosages.

Furthermore, capsules are portable and discreet. If you need to take your herbs while at work or traveling, carrying a bottle of capsules is much more convenient than taking along bags of loose herbs. You can easily incorporate them into your daily routine without drawing too much attention.

Lastly, encapsulating herbs can help preserve their freshness. The capsule forms a barrier that protects the herb from air and moisture, two factors that can accelerate the degradation process and decrease potency. Therefore, encapsulating herbs can extend their shelf life, ensuring you get the most out of your herbal investment.

Step-By-Step Guide to Encapsulating Herbs

A step-by-step guide to encapsulating herbs can make the process much easier, especially for those new to the practice. Here, we will walk through the basic steps for encapsulating Dr. Sebi's herbs:

<u>Measure the Herbs</u>: Begin by measuring out the quantity of ground herbs you want to encapsulate. Each 00-sized capsule typically holds about 500 mg of herbs, so plan accordingly based on your desired dosage.

<u>Prepare the Capsules</u>: Purchase empty capsules from a health food store or online. They often come in two parts: a larger bottom piece (the "body") and a smaller top piece (the "cap"). Separate the two halves of the capsules.

<u>Fill the Capsules</u>: Scoop up some of your ground herbs with the body of the capsule. Fill it as much as you can without spilling over.

<u>Cap the Capsules</u>: Once the body of the capsule is filled with herbs, take the cap and press it onto the body until it clicks into place.

<u>Store the Capsules</u>: Place your completed capsules in a clean, airtight container. Store the container in a cool, dry place away from sunlight.

<u>Clean Up</u>: Ensure you clean all your equipment thoroughly after each use to avoid cross-contamination between different herbs.

Remember that these are general steps and might need slight adjustments depending on the type of capsule machine you are using or the specific herbs you are encapsulating. Always follow any instructions provided with your capsule machine or the capsules themselves.

Materials Required for Encapsulation

As with any DIY process, having the right materials at hand is crucial for successful encapsulation of herbs. Here is a list of materials you'll need when encapsulating Dr. Sebi's herbs:

Herb Grinder: A good-quality herb grinder is essential. It ensures your herbs are finely ground for easy absorption and fitting into capsules.

Scale: To measure out your herbs accurately, a precise scale is necessary. This is particularly important if you're aiming to achieve a specific dosage with each capsule.

Empty Capsules: These are available in various sizes, with 00 being the most common for herbal supplementation. You can find them in most health food stores or online. They're often made from gelatin or a vegetarian alternative like HPMC.

Capsule Filling Machine: While not absolutely necessary, a capsule filling machine can greatly speed up the process, especially if you plan on making large quantities. They hold the capsule bodies in place, allowing you to fill numerous capsules at once.

<u>Funnel or Tray</u>: If you don't have a capsule filling machine, a small funnel or a specially designed tray can help direct the ground herbs into the capsule bodies without spilling.

<u>Clean Containers</u>: You will need clean, airtight containers to store your finished capsules. Glass jars work well for this purpose.

Remember, quality matters. Using high-quality materials and tools will not only make the process smoother but also ensure the purity and potency of your herbal capsules.

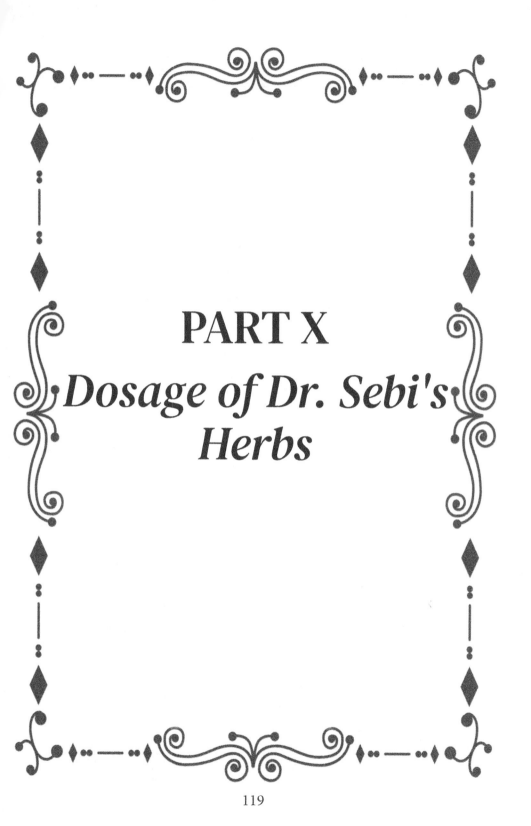

PART X
Dosage of Dr. Sebi's Herbs

BONUS EXTRA!!!

Scan the QR CODE

and Get Your Free Digital Full-Color Edition of **Dr. Sebi's 7-Day Full-Body Detox Plan** and **Dr. Sebi's Alkaline Herbs Guide** to Recognize the Herbs while Harvesting them Yourself - All Straight into Your Email!!

As SPAM Filters Are Pretty Crazy These Days...
...WHITELIST this Email Address!

info@greenessencepublishing.com

In This Way, Your Bonus Will Appear in the Main Folder of Your INBOX and They Will Not Be Buried Along With Other Advertisements in Your PROMOTION/SPAM Folder.

HERE IS HOW TO DO IT:
From Android Smartphone/Tablet
Open the Contacts App;
In the lower right corner, tap + (Add);
Enter the name and email address and then tap Save.

From iPhone/iPad
Open the Contacts App;
In the upper right corner, tap + (Add);
Enter the name and email address and then tap Finish.

Understanding Dosage

When talking about herbal medicine and Dr. Sebi's herbs, understanding dosage is essential. Dosage refers to the amount of a substance, in this case, a medicinal herb, to be consumed within a specific period, often denoted as a certain quantity per day.

The importance of understanding and adhering to the recommended dosage cannot be overstated. The effectiveness of an herb is closely tied to the dosage taken - both under-dosing and overdosing can lead to suboptimal results or potential adverse effects.

Under-dosing can result in not achieving the desired therapeutic effect. It's like trying to fill up a bath tub with a trickle of water - it's unlikely to be effective. On the other hand, taking too high a dose, or overdosing, may increase the risk of potential side effects. It may be too much for your body to handle all at once, akin to attempting to quench your thirst by drinking from a fire hose.

Additionally, different herbs have different potency levels. Some are highly potent and require only minute doses to exert their effects, while others might need to be taken in larger quantities. It's crucial to research and understand the dosage requirements for each specific herb you plan on incorporating into your health regimen.

In the next section, we will look into how to determine the correct dosage for Dr. Sebi's herbs.

How to Determine Correct Dosage

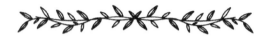

Determining the correct dosage of Dr. Sebi's herbs involves several factors. Each individual is unique, and what works for one person might not work for another. The factors that come into play when determining dosage include age, weight, overall health status, and the specific health concern being addressed.

Age: Generally, adults can tolerate larger doses than children. This is not only due to body size but also to the maturity of bodily systems, including the liver and kidneys, which play significant roles in metabolizing substances and eliminating waste products from the body.

Weight: Dosage is often determined in relation to a person's weight. Someone who weighs more will usually require a larger dose than someone who weighs less.

Overall health status: People who are generally healthy might tolerate higher doses of herbs better than those who are not. People with compromised liver or kidney function, or with other serious health conditions, may need to adjust dosages accordingly and should do so under the supervision of a healthcare professional familiar with herbal medicine.

Specific health concern: The dosage may also depend on the specific health concern. For example, a condition that is chronic or severe might require a higher dose than a minor or acute condition.

The herb's potency: Some herbs are more potent than others. An herb that is highly potent will require a smaller dose than an herb that is less potent.

It's important to start with a smaller dose and gradually increase it, observing your body's reactions, until you reach a dose that is effective for you. It's also beneficial to keep a journal noting the doses taken and your body's responses. This can be very helpful in fine-tuning your dosage.

In the next section, we'll explore guidelines for adjusting dosages over time.

Guidelines for Adjusting Dosages Over Time

Adjusting the dosage of Dr. Sebi's herbs over time is an integral part of their effective use. As you use these herbal remedies, your body's responses can change, which may necessitate adjusting the dosage.

Body's Response: Keep a close eye on your body's response to the herbal remedy. If you notice any adverse reactions, such as nausea, vomiting, headaches, or other unusual symptoms, it's a clear indication that you need to adjust your dosage. This may mean reducing it until the adverse reactions subside.

Effectiveness: If, after using a specific dose for a certain period, you observe that the remedy's effectiveness has lessened, you might need to increase the dosage slightly. Always increase the dosage gradually and never exceed the recommended maximum dose.

Health Improvement: If your health condition improves considerably, you may need to decrease the dosage or even stop taking the herb entirely. For instance, if your blood pressure levels stabilize after using a particular herb, it would be wise to lower the dosage under the guidance of a healthcare professional.

Long-term use: Some herbs can have diminishing effects if used over a long time at the same dosage. In such cases, you may need to increase the dose slightly. However, it's essential to take breaks to prevent the body from getting too accustomed to the herb, leading to reduced effectiveness.

Professional Guidance: Consulting with a healthcare professional familiar with Dr. Sebi's herbs is always recommended when adjusting dosages. They can provide guidance based on your specific health conditions and responses to the herbs.

Remember, the goal of using Dr. Sebi's herbs is to achieve optimal health, and sometimes, adjusting the dosage is necessary to reach this goal. Use your own judgment and listen to your body; it will often tell you what it needs.

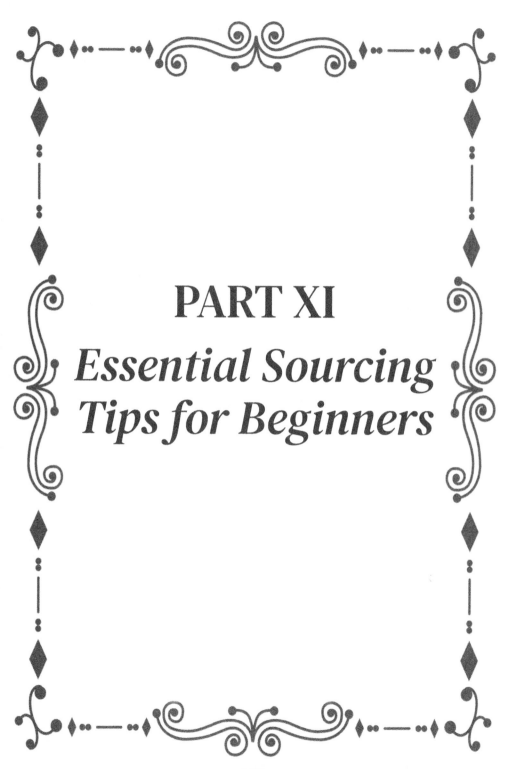

PART XI
Essential Sourcing Tips for Beginners

Building Relationships with Trusted Suppliers

Building strong relationships with trusted suppliers is a journey in itself, an invaluable aspect of sourcing Dr. Sebi's herbs. The security and consistency that comes with having a reliable and reputable supplier ensures access to high-quality, organic, and wildcrafted herbs that are in line with Dr. Sebi's principles.

This bond, though it may seem challenging to establish at first, is built over time. Its foundations are set on trust, regular communication, and a shared commitment to integrity. Initial steps include carrying out thorough research to understand the ethical and sustainable sourcing methods employed by the supplier. It's crucial to identify suppliers who prioritize organic, wildcrafted, or naturally grown herbs.

Once you've identified potential suppliers, fostering open and frequent communication is vital. Establishing a dialogue allows for an understanding of the supplier's processes and also demonstrates your interest in their work. As your relationship strengthens over time, the mutual trust that develops can open doors to exclusive deals, insider knowledge, and a dependable supply of high-quality herbs.

Understanding Market Prices for Herbs

Understanding the market prices for herbs is a crucial element of successful sourcing. It not only helps ensure you're paying a fair price, but also helps protect against fraud and exploitation.

The market price for herbs fluctuates due to numerous factors, including the time of year, environmental conditions, and the quality of the herbs. It's important to stay informed about these dynamics. Knowing the average prices for specific herbs helps to make informed buying decisions and negotiate with confidence.

It is also worth noting that prices for organic, wildcrafted, and sustainably sourced herbs are often higher than their conventionally grown counterparts. This price difference reflects the higher costs associated with these more responsible cultivation methods, but it's often a worthwhile investment for the superior quality, potency, and environmental benefits they offer.

Lastly, remember that price should not be your only consideration. The quality, sustainability, and ethical considerations associated with sourcing herbs should be as much a priority as cost.

Tips for Avoiding Common Sourcing Mistakes

As a beginner in the world of sourcing Dr. Sebi's herbs, you might face certain challenges and make mistakes. This is a natural part of the learning process, and these pitfalls can be avoided with a bit of foresight and preparation.

One common mistake is not thoroughly vetting suppliers. Remember, not every supplier who claims to provide organic or wildcrafted herbs is legitimate. Do your homework and ensure the supplier has a solid reputation, provides transparency about their sourcing practices, and adheres to high-quality standards.

Next, be aware of the temptation to opt for the cheapest option. While it might seem like a good idea to save money, lower-priced herbs often come at the cost of lower quality, adulteration, or unethical sourcing practices. Your priority should always be quality and sustainability over price.

Also, be sure to understand the natural growing seasons of the herbs you're sourcing. Out-of-season herbs may have been stored for long periods, which can lead to a decrease in potency.

By avoiding these common mistakes, you'll be well on your way to successfully sourcing Dr. Sebi's herbs and reaping the incredible health benefits they offer.

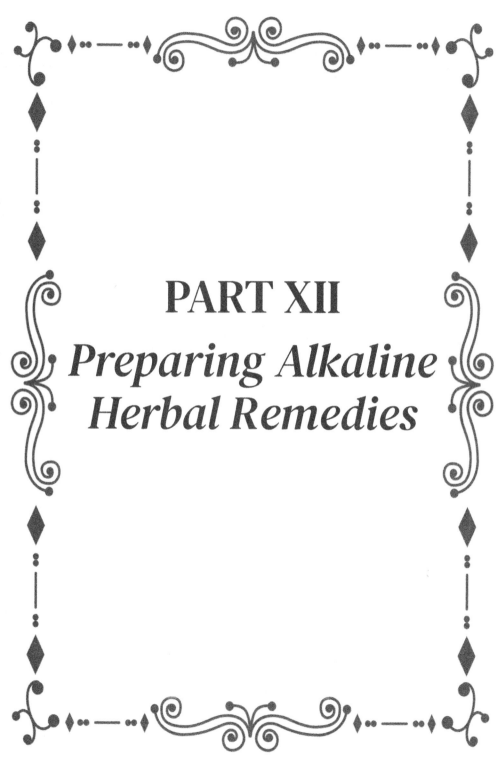

PART XII
Preparing Alkaline Herbal Remedies

Preparing Herbal Teas for Detoxification and Healing

Herbal teas are a soothing and simple way to absorb the benefits of alkaline herbs. These teas can be enjoyed throughout the day, and with the right combination of herbs, they can play a significant role in detoxification and healing. Here, we'll explore how to prepare herbal teas using Dr. Sebi's approved alkaline herbs.

Basic Steps for Preparing Herbal Tea

<u>Choose Your Herbs</u>: Depending on your specific health concerns or detoxification needs, you may wish to choose different combinations of herbs. For example, you might select burdock root and elderberry for immune support or sarsaparilla for its antioxidant properties.

<u>Measure Your Herbs</u>: A good rule of thumb is to use one teaspoon of dried herb or one tablespoon of fresh herb per cup of water. If you're combining herbs, adjust the quantity of each accordingly.

<u>Heat Your Water</u>: Bring your water to a boil in a non-reactive pot, such as a stainless steel or glass pot. Avoid aluminum or non-stick surfaces.

<u>Add Your Herbs</u>: Once the water is boiling, add your herbs. Stir them in to ensure they're fully immersed in the water.

<u>Simmer or Steep</u>: If you're making a simple infusion (suitable for more delicate parts of the plant like leaves or flowers), turn off the heat and let your herbs steep for 15 to 20 minutes. If you're using tougher plant parts (like roots or barks) in a decoction, reduce the heat to a simmer and let the herbs steep for longer, usually about 20-30 minutes.

<u>Strain and Serve</u>: After the appropriate steeping time, strain the herbs out of the water using a fine mesh strainer. Your tea is now ready to enjoy! If desired, you can sweeten it with a natural sweetener like agave syrup but remember that part of Dr. Sebi's approach includes reducing processed sugars.

Herbal teas are a staple in the alkaline diet advocated by Dr. Sebi. They are a simple yet effective way to benefit from the healing and detoxifying properties of alkaline herbs. Enjoy them hot or cold, and experiment with different combinations to find the mix that works best for your individual health needs.

Crafting Infusions for Enhanced Wellbeing

Herbal infusions are a slightly more concentrated form of herbal tea. They involve steeping a larger amount of herb in water for a longer period of time, allowing for more nutrients to be extracted. These potent brews are an excellent way to target specific health concerns or simply promote overall wellbeing. Let's delve into the process of crafting your own alkaline herbal infusions.

Before beginning, always ensure you're using quality herbs—organic, wildcrafted, or sustainably sourced. Always consult with a healthcare provider before starting a new herbal regimen, especially if you're pregnant, nursing, or have any chronic health conditions.

How to Prepare Herbal Infusions

<u>Select Your Herbs</u>: As with herbal teas, you'll want to choose your herbs based on your individual health needs or desired outcomes. An infusion made with bladderwrack (Fucus vesiculosus) and sea moss (Chondrus crispus) could be beneficial for thyroid support, while burdock root (Arctium lappa) might be chosen for its blood-cleansing properties.

Measure Your Herbs: For an infusion, you'll typically want to use a larger quantity of herbs than you would for a tea. One common ratio is one ounce of dried herb (or one and a half ounces of fresh herb) per quart of water.

Add Herbs to a Jar: Place your herbs in a clean, quart-sized glass jar.

Boil Water: Bring a quart of water to a boil.

Pour Over Herbs: Pour the boiling water over your herbs in the jar, filling it to the top.

Steep: Cover the jar, and let your herbs steep for a minimum of four hours, but ideally overnight. This long steeping time allows for a maximum extraction of the beneficial compounds in the herbs.

Strain: After steeping, strain the infusion using a fine-mesh strainer or cheesecloth. Discard or compost the used herbs.

Store and Serve: Store your infusion in the refrigerator, where it will keep for several days. You can drink it cold or gently warmed, and it can be consumed on its own or added to smoothies, juices, or other recipes.

Crafting your own herbal infusions can be a rewarding way to enhance your wellbeing and deepen your relationship with Dr. Sebi's approved alkaline herbs. Infusions allow for a greater extraction of nutrients, offering a potent and flavorful way to support your health.

Creating Decoctions for Targeted Health Concerns

A decoction is yet another method of extracting the beneficial properties from herbs. Unlike infusions which are typically used for more delicate plant parts like leaves and flowers, decoctions are specifically designed for tougher materials such as roots, barks, seeds and berries. In this chapter, we'll discuss the process of creating alkaline herbal decoctions for targeted health concerns using Dr. Sebi's approved herbs.

How to Prepare Herbal Decoctions

<u>Choose Your Herbs</u>: As with teas and infusions, you'll select your herbs based on your health needs. For instance, a decoction of sarsaparilla root (Smilax ornata) could be beneficial for joint pain, while yellow dock root (Rumex crispus) might be employed for its liver-supportive properties.

<u>Measure Your Herbs</u>: Typically, you'll want to use about one ounce of dried herb for each quart of water, but this can vary depending on the specific herb and your individual needs.

<u>Combine Herbs and Water</u>: Unlike an infusion where boiling water is poured over the herbs, in a decoction, the herbs and water are added to the pot together.

<u>Simmer</u>: Bring your pot to a boil, then reduce the heat to a low simmer. Allow your herbs to simmer for approximately 20-30 minutes. This heat and time combination helps to extract the beneficial compounds from the tougher plant materials.

<u>Strain</u>: After simmering, strain the decoction into a glass or jar, being sure to press or squeeze the herbs to extract as much liquid as possible. Discard the used herbs.

<u>Store and Serve</u>: Store your decoction in the refrigerator. It should be consumed within a few days for maximum freshness and potency. Decoctions can be consumed on their own, or they can be added to other beverages or recipes.

Through decoctions, you can tap into the deep, nourishing properties of Dr. Sebi's approved alkaline herbs. This method provides a concentrated dose of plant power, offering a targeted approach to address specific health concerns.

Mastering The Art of Mixing Dr. Sebi's Herbs for Healing

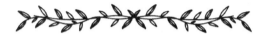

Combining Dr. Sebi's approved herbs for healing is an art steeped in understanding and respect for the unique qualities of each herb. This process is about achieving balance and synergy that can result in a more potent and customized healing solution.

The foundations of effective herbal blending hinge on recognizing the individual strengths, properties, and healing potentials of each herb. For instance, some herbs may act as relaxants, while others can energize and stimulate. Knowing these specific traits will guide you in creating a mix that serves your unique needs.

Furthermore, certain herbs, when combined, can enhance one another's medicinal properties - a synergy that can create a more powerful healing effect than when used separately. Contrarily, others may interfere with each other's functions, neutralizing their benefits or causing unwanted side effects. As such, understanding these interplays is vital in designing your personalized herbal combinations.

Creating Therapeutic Herbal Blends:

Immune Boosting Blend: A combination of elderberry, which is known for its immune-enhancing properties, with red clover and burdock root, both recognized as blood purifiers, may provide a helpful blend for immune support.

Brain Health Blend: For enhancing mental clarity and supporting brain health, mixing herbs like chamomile with its soothing effect and the nervine properties of blue vervain might be beneficial.

Digestive Support Blend: A mix of prodijiosa, known for supporting digestive health, with the liver-supporting properties of dandelion root and the stomach-soothing properties of chamomile, may help create a well-rounded digestive blend.

Energy and Vitality Blend: For an energizing mix, consider blending the iron-rich yellow dock and sarsaparilla, known for its tonifying properties, with the energizing effects of Irish sea moss, which is loaded with beneficial nutrients.

Relaxation Blend: For a calming and sleep-supporting blend, combining the relaxing properties of valerian root and tila, with the soothing effects of chamomile, can create a mix that may aid restful sleep and relaxation.

Skin Health Blend: Bladderwrack, rich in skin-supporting minerals, mixed with the detoxifying properties of burdock root and the skin-soothing attributes of chamomile might be beneficial for skin health.

Remember, it's always important to start with small doses when experimenting with new blends, and to monitor your body's responses closely.

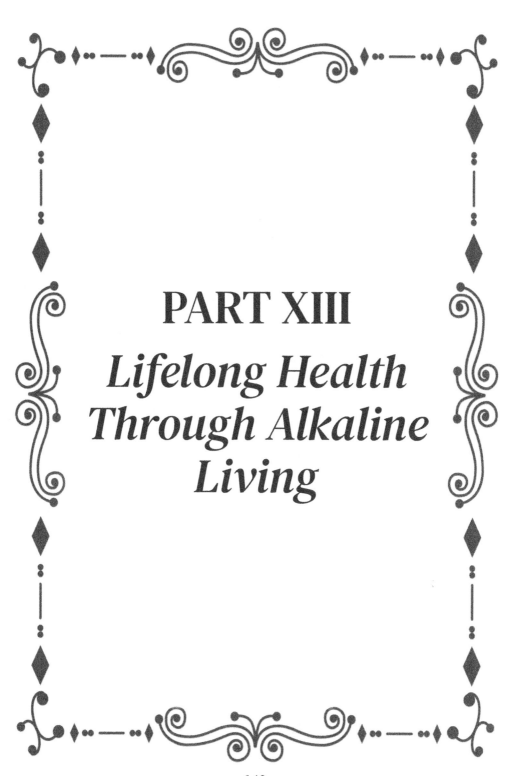

PART XIII
Lifelong Health Through Alkaline Living

Integrating Alkaline Herbs into Your Daily Life

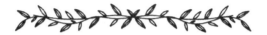

Embracing an alkaline lifestyle means more than just an occasional cleanse or detoxification regimen. It involves integrating the principles and practices into your daily life, and herbs play an important role in this.

1. Morning Rituals:

Start your day with an alkaline boost. You could begin your day with an herbal tea such as burdock root (Arctium lappa) or bladderwrack (Fucus vesiculosus) which can be beneficial in kickstarting your metabolism and detoxification for the day.

2. Cooking with Herbs:

Cooking with alkaline herbs can transform your meals into healing remedies. Add fresh or dried herbs to your meals for added flavor and health benefits. For example, sea moss (Chondrus crispus), a Dr. Sebi-approved herb, can be used as a nutrient-rich thickening agent in soups, stews, and sauces.

3. Herbal Supplements:

Consider supplementing your diet with alkaline herbs in capsule form. Capsules can provide a convenient way to incorporate the benefits of these herbs, especially when you're on the go. Herbs like bladderwrack, sea moss, and sarsaparilla are often available in capsule form.

4. Creating a Herbal Sanctuary at Home:

You may also consider growing your own herbs at home. This could be as simple as a windowsill garden or as extensive as an outdoor herbal plot. Growing your own herbs can offer a deeper connection to these plants, not to mention the convenience and cost savings.

5. Evening Rituals:

Ending your day with a soothing herbal tea like chamomile promote restful sleep and relaxation.

Integrating alkaline herbs into your daily routine doesn't have to be complex or time-consuming. With a bit of planning and creativity, you can easily weave these powerful plants into your everyday life, bringing you closer to optimal health and wellbeing. Remember, consistency is key when it comes to experiencing the full benefits of alkaline herbs.

Alkaline Diet: Complementing Herbal Intake

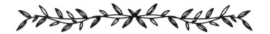

Incorporating alkaline herbs into your daily life can offer a host of health benefits, from detoxification to rejuvenation. However, to maximize these benefits, it's crucial to complement your herbal intake with a wholesome alkaline diet. Here's how you can create a balanced alkaline eating plan that harmonizes with your alkaline herbal regimen:

1. Embrace Plant-Based Foods:

An alkaline diet primarily focuses on plant-based foods, which are naturally high in alkaline minerals such as calcium, magnesium, and potassium. Fill your plate with fresh vegetables, fruits, legumes, nuts, and seeds. Foods such as avocados, cucumbers, lime, bell peppers, and quinoa are excellent alkaline choices.

2. Limit Acid-Forming Foods:

While maintaining an alkaline diet, it's important to limit the intake of acid-forming foods. This includes processed foods, refined sugars, dairy products, meat, and certain grains. While it may seem challenging at first, with time, you'll find that your taste buds and body start to crave alkaline foods.

3. *Hydrate:*

Hydration is essential in an alkaline diet. Drink plenty of water and infuse it with alkalizing herbs added benefits.

4. *Pairing Foods:*

Certain food combinations can improve absorption of nutrients and contribute to an alkaline balance. Pairing iron-rich foods like spinach with vitamin C-rich foods like bell peppers can enhance iron absorption.

5. *Listen to Your Body:*

Everyone's body reacts differently to dietary changes. Pay attention to how your body responds as you transition to an alkaline diet. If certain foods don't agree with you, it's important to adjust your diet accordingly.

By adhering to an alkaline diet, you're providing your body with the nutrient-dense, alkalizing foods it needs to support and enhance the benefits of your alkaline herbal regimen. Combined, these practices can pave the way for long-term health and vitality.

Long-Term Maintenance of Health: Tips and Tricks

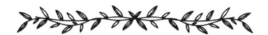

Embracing the alkaline lifestyle is about much more than following a temporary diet or herbal regimen. It's about committing to a way of life that fosters lifelong health and vitality. As you continue your journey towards optimal health with alkaline herbs and diet, here are a few tips and tricks for long-term maintenance of health:

1. Regular Exercise:

Movement is vital for maintaining overall health. Engaging in regular physical activity not only helps balance your pH levels but also enhances your mood, boosts energy levels, and supports cardiovascular health. Choose a form of exercise that you enjoy, whether that's walking, yoga, swimming, or cycling.

2. Mindful Eating:

Tuning in to your body's signals can significantly enhance your health. Practice mindful eating by paying attention to your hunger and fullness cues. Take time to appreciate your meals, savoring each bite and acknowledging the nourishment you are providing your body.

3. Consistent Herbal Intake:

Consistency is key when it comes to the benefits of alkaline herbs. Make herbal infusions, teas, and decoctions a regular part of your daily routine. Remember, the transformative power of these herbs builds over time with consistent use.

4. Embrace Variety:

To ensure you're receiving a wide range of nutrients, aim for variety in both your diet and herbal regimen. Rotate between different alkaline foods and herbs to maintain balance and keep your meals exciting.

5. Regular Check-ups:

Regular health check-ups can provide useful insights into your body's needs and the progress of your alkaline journey. This, in combination with awareness of how you feel, can help you tailor your diet and herbal intake more effectively.

6. Stress Management:

Chronic stress can disrupt your body's balance, leading to various health problems. Incorporate stress-reducing activities into your routine, such as meditation, deep breathing exercises, or spending time in nature.

Remember, the journey to lifelong health is a marathon, not a sprint. Be patient with yourself and celebrate your progress along the way. By making these habits a part of your everyday life, you're setting the stage for long-term health and vitality.

APPENDIX A:
Frequently Asked
Questions

In this section, we aim to address some of the most common questions that arise when one embarks on the journey of alkaline living and the use of Dr. Sebi approved herbs.

1. Can I use more than one herb at a time?

Yes, many of Dr. Sebi's herbal formulas contain multiple herbs that work synergistically to deliver greater benefits. However, if you're new to herbal therapy, it's wise to start with one herb at a time to monitor how your body reacts.

2. How long will it take to see results from using alkaline herbs?

The timeline for results can vary widely depending on individual factors such as the current state of health, consistency of use, diet, and lifestyle habits. Some people experience noticeable improvements within weeks, while for others, it may take months.

3. Can I take alkaline herbs while pregnant or breastfeeding?

Some alkaline herbs are safe to use during pregnancy and breastfeeding, but others are not. Always consult with a healthcare professional before starting any new herbal regimen during these periods.

4. Can children use alkaline herbs?

Most alkaline herbs are safe for children in appropriate doses, but always consult with a pediatrician or herbalist experienced in pediatric care before giving herbs to children.

5. Can I use alkaline herbs if I'm taking medication?

It's important to consult with your healthcare provider before starting any herbal regimen if you're currently taking medication. Some herbs can interact with medications, potentially causing adverse effects.

6. Where can I buy alkaline herbs?

There are various online and physical stores where you can purchase alkaline herbs. Please see the next section on 'Resources for Purchasing High-Quality Alkaline Herbs' for recommendations.

This FAQ section addresses the most common inquiries we receive about alkaline herbs and the alkaline lifestyle. However, it's crucial to remember that everyone's journey is unique. Your path to optimal health will be shaped by your individual experiences, and there is no 'one-size-fits-all' answer. Be patient, stay consistent, and always listen to your body.